Art Therapy Directives

T0372892

Art Therapy Directives: An Intervention Toolbox is an all-inclusive manual of art therapy directives designed to be a comprehensive and organized resource for art therapists and other trained mental health professionals. Art therapy directives are directions for creating art and often require the use of specific art media, both of which are tailored to the client's particular needs. Using this book, art therapists will be able to search by population, themes, and art media to find just the right project for their session, whether working with individuals or in groups. Comprised of a compilation of traditional art therapy directives, the author's own experiences, and other published practices, a wide range of mental health topics are included, such as depression, self-esteem, life transitions, and trauma. Special consideration is given to populations like adolescents, older adults, veterans, and the LGBTQIA+ community. This manual is the answer that many in the field of art therapy have been missing for an all-encompassing, organized reference book to guide art therapy sessions with a wide variety of client populations.

Sarah Balascio is a nationally board-certified art therapist and adjunct lecturer with over 15 years of experience working with children, adolescents, adults, seniors, families, and groups. Currently, she works at the College of William & Mary's McLeod Tyler Wellness Center, facilitating groups and individual sessions for students, faculty, and staff, as well as teaching undergraduate courses in the field of art therapy under the Wellness Applications Program. She also serves on the Art Therapy Credentials Board Nominating Committee.

"*Art Therapy Directives: An Intervention Toolbox* offers the field of art therapy a much-needed resource for those who use the creative arts therapies with clients. I highly recommend this book for anyone who wants intervention ideas and practical 'how-to' guides for growth and healing. It includes all the art mediums and pertinent clinical issues in a variety of settings. This is the most comprehensive resource I have come across."

Allison Crowe, PhD, LCMHC-S *Professor, Counselor Education, Interim Department Chair, Interdisciplinary Professions, East Carolina University*

"A prominent place on every art therapist's bookshelves should be reserved for the innovative book *Art Therapy Directives: An Intervention Toolbox*. This book serves as a thorough guide delivering inspiration and real-world applications to address a wide range of therapeutic interventions thanks to its extensive yet thorough examination of the subject matter by the author Sarah Balascio. An excellent tool for art therapists seeking to advance their practice and ultimately aid in the healing of their clients, it is filled with the author's broad knowledge and professional experience."

Cheryl Walpole Tiku MPS, LPC, LCAT, LPAT, ATR-BC, *Licensed Professional Counselor, Licensed Creative Arts Therapist, Texas, New York, New Jersey*

"I have had the fortunate opportunity to witness first hand the transformational and healing impact of Sarah's work on our campus. I'm so excited that Sarah has taken on the task of sharing her talents with a broader audience through this very well-written and creatively organized book *Art Therapy Directives: An Intervention Toolbox*. I am admiring and impressed in how she not only provided a flexible reference guide for fellow art therapists and students in art therapy, but she has done a masterful job of revealing the profession of art therapy. As a mental health professional, but not an art therapist, who has witnessed the impact of her work, I gained a glimpse into the process of her work and why expressive therapies are curative and corrective in people's lives. She found the perfect balance of providing clear, easily referenced guidance to multiple therapeutic themes along the entire neurodiverse continuum with relevant therapeutic directives, while being very clear that it is not a template to be followed without consideration of the art therapists themselves and their clients. She accomplished what is most difficult about therapeutic texts, taking the complex relational dynamics of therapy and translating why she is so effective into book form that others can effectively utilize. I was left with a deeper appreciation and value of art therapy that was already very high, and an excitement about this invaluable contribution to the field."

R. Kelly Crace, PhD, *Associate Vice President for Health & Wellness, Director, Center for Mindfulness & Authentic Excellence (CMAX)*

Art Therapy Directives

An Intervention Toolbox

Sarah Balascio

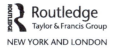
Routledge
Taylor & Francis Group

NEW YORK AND LONDON

Cover image: © Getty Images

First published 2024
by Routledge
605 Third Avenue, New York, NY 10158

and by Routledge
4 Park Square, Milton Park, Abingdon, Oxon, OX14 4RN

*Routledge is an imprint of the Taylor & Francis Group, an informa
business*

© 2024 Sarah Balascio

The right Sarah Balascio to be identified as author of this work
has been asserted in accordance with sections 77 and 78 of the
Copyright, Designs and Patents Act 1988.

ISBN: 978-1-032-53740-5 (hbk)
ISBN: 978-1-032-53739-9 (pbk)
ISBN: 978-1-003-41336-3 (ebk)

DOI: 10.4324/9781003413363

Typeset in Times New Roman
by KnowledgeWorks Global Ltd.

Access the Support Material: www.routledge.com/9781032537399

This book is dedicated to the loves of my life
Nick, Will, and Drew
and for those who have struggled with mental health
and been courageous enough to seek help.

Contents

List of Images   ix
About the Author   xi
Acknowledgments   xii
List of Abbreviations   xiv

1 Introduction   1

2 Adolescents and Young Adults   10

3 Anger Management   15

4 Anxiety   18

5 Autism Spectrum Disorder   22

6 Children   26

7 Depression   30

8 Eating Disorders   34

9 Eco-Art   38

10 Emotion Recognition   43

11 Families   47

12 Grief   50

13 Group Rapport   54

14 LGBTQIA+   58

15 Life Transitions   62

16 Medical Art Therapy   67

17 Mindfulness   72

18 Multiculturalism   77

19 Older Adults and Dementia   82

20 Personality Disorders   86

21 Pregnancy, Infertility, and Women's Health   90

22 Psychotic Disorders   94

23 Self-Esteem   97

24 Spirituality   101

25 Substance Abuse and Addiction   105

26 Supervision   109

27 Termination   113

28 Trauma   117

29 Veterans & First Responders   121

30 Warm Ups & Creative Exploration   125

31 Virtual Art Therapy   130

32 Conclusion   133

    Index   *136*

Images

2.1	Secret Word Mandala (Folded)	12
2.2	Secret Word Mandala (Completed)	13
3.1	Collaborative Anger Sculpture	17
4.1	Lavender Eye Pillow	20
5.1	Pillow Stuffed Animal	23
5.2	Paper Quilling Examples	24
6.1	Power Word Jewelry	28
7.1	Gratitude Tree Watercolor	32
8.1	Clay Image of "Ed".	35
8.2	Charcoal Drawing of Recovery Dialectics: *Fear of Change and Wanting to Recover*	36
9.1	Collaborative Eco-Art Sculpture	39
9.2	Rock Wrapping	41
10.1	Painting of Anxiety	45
11.1	Collaborative Painting	48
12.1	Letting Go Leaf (with Template)	51
12.2	Letting Go Leaf	52
13.1	Group Art Making	55
14.1	Pride Button	59
15.1	*"I Come From"* Art Journaling Example	65
16.1	Finger Knitting	70
17.1	Mind-Full versus Mindful Drawing	74
17.2	Zendoodle® Landscape Example	75
18.1	Heritage Square Fiber Art	78
18.2	Piece of Me Mixed Media Technique	80
19.1	Simple Sock Doll Making	84
20.1	Decorative Diary Card	87
21.1	Clay Imprints	91

21.2	Nest Examples	92
22.1	Watercolor Abstract	96
23.1	Affirmation Word Watercolor	98
24.1	Heart and Soul Watercolor	102
25.1	Plaster Safe Haven (in Progress)	107
26.1	Chakras Watercolor Reflection	110
27.1	Gateway Drawing	114
28.1	Clay Soothing Stone	119
29.1	Art Journaling Example	122
29.2	Shame Off You Drawing	124
30.1	Finish This Drawing Example Starter Line	126
30.2	Paper Mache Mask Examples	127

About the Author

Sarah Balascio is a nationally board-certified art therapist and adjunct lecturer with over 15 years of experience working with children, adolescents, adults, seniors, families, and groups. Sarah has a master's degree in Education from Lesley University in Massachusetts and a second master's degree in Art Therapy from Pratt Institute in New York. She has practiced art therapy in hospitals, including New York Presbyterian, residential programs for adolescents, eating disorder treatment centers, schools, autism centers, and in private practice. She has helped clients with issues such as anxiety, depression, life transitions, eating disorders, trauma, grief, addictions, developmental, and sensory issues, as well as autism spectrum disorders. She now works at the College of William & Mary's McLeod Tyler Wellness Center, facilitating groups and individual sessions for students, faculty, and staff, as well as teaching undergraduate courses in the field of art therapy under the Wellness Applications Program. She also serves on the Art Therapy Credentials Board Nominating Committee.

Acknowledgments

There are a number of people to thank for helping with this book. Most importantly, I would like to thank all of the clients, patients, residents, families, group members, and students who have been a part of my work and who make me love my job as an art therapist every day. I would next like to thank my publisher, Routledge Taylor & Francis, and in particular my Editor, Amanda Savage and Editorial Assistant(s), Katya Porter and Priya Sharma. I would also like to thank the peer reviewers who donated their time and thoughts and most definitely made this book better. In particular, thank you to Cheryl Walpole Tiku, a friend, fellow Pratt alum, and New York Presbyterian colleague. I would also like to acknowledge my art therapy graduate degree from Pratt Institute that I consider life-changing. Along the same lines, I am so grateful for my educational, internship, and professional supervisors throughout my career path.

The idea for this book came out of a post on Art Therapy Online, a professional social media group for art therapists. A fellow art therapist, Kate Colson, asked for something like this as a resource, which spurred this idea. I hope it is helpful two years later.

At the College of William & Mary, I would like to thank my supervisors at the McLeod Tyler Wellness Center, Kelly Crace and Lindsay Heck, for their true understanding and appreciation of the field of art therapy. A special thank you to Lindsay for the photography help. I would also like to acknowledge Raven Pierce, a student mentee who I know will do great things in the field of mental health. I would like to thank Liz Cascone at The Haven and Julie Cullifer at One Child Center for Autism for their collaboration and expertise in their professional areas.

I owe a special thank you to Allison Smith Crowe, Professor and Interim Department Chair at East Carolina University. Not only are you my best friend, but you are also a brilliant colleague. Thank you for all your advising and brainstorming. I would also like to thank my sisterhood: Andrea, Caitlin, Jen, Kara, Kelly, Meg, Myndi, Nicole, and Sara. These are the types of women you can call in the middle of the night or who call you with the chills because you just typed your last word of your book. While writing this book in Norway, I had a special writing partner, Cate Fricke, who kept me focused while we hopped from café to café. I would also like to thank Akiko and Yuki for their assistance as we sat fjord side in Lofthus, Norway.

Last but not least, I would like to thank my husband Nick and my sons Will and Drew Balascio for their support along the way. Nick you have instilled a confidence in me that I may not always know is there, and you suggest wild adventures like living in a foreign country for a year and writing a book! I love you for that.

Abbreviations

AA	Alcoholics Anonymous
AATA	American Art Therapy Association
ACT	Acceptance and Commitment Therapy
AD	Alzheimer's Disease
ASD	Autism Spectrum Disorder
ATCB	Art Therapy Credentials Board
ATCS	Art Therapy Credentialed Supervisor
ATR	Registered Art Therapist
ATR-BC	Registered Art Therapist – Board Certified
ATR-P	Registered Art Therapist – Provisional
BPD	Borderline Personality Disorder
CBT	Cognitive Behavioral Therapy
DBT	Dialectical Behavior Therapy
DMT	Dance Movement Therapist
ED	Eating Disorder
LGBTQIA+	Lesbian, Gay, Bisexual, Transgender, Queer, Intersex, Asexual, Plus
NA	Narcotics Anonymous
PTSD	Post Traumatic Stress Disorder
SMART	Self Management and Recovery Training

Chapter 1

Introduction

As my family and I prepared for a year abroad in Bergen, Norway, on sabbatical, with a greatly reduced work schedule, I wondered aloud to my husband what I should do with my time there? Sure, I would help my children acclimate and do more of my own art, but knowing myself I would need more than that. My husband, who is an associate professor in Geology, suggested writing a book that I had had in the back of my mind for a couple of years. The idea sounded so romantic, hopping from café to café in rainy Bergen, Norway, trying various cappuccinos with my trusty laptop in tow. Yes, this was partially true, but writing a book is so hard! I now have a new found appreciation for any author. Also, sorry to offend Norwegians, but your coffee is dreadful! The year abroad was life-changing and writing this book has been too. The idea was formed through my art therapy community, one of which I am so proud to be a part of. I was reading through an art therapy social media group, and I noticed a peer asked the group for a compilation of art therapy directives. While originally more casual, she even asked for paper files, but I thought this would make a great book. I thought to myself that I could use this too. There were some book recommendations tossed around in the comments, but none that were more of a reference style with a wide variety of different topics and populations. There are also so many well-written in-depth books about various populations or specific issues within the field of art therapy. I thought to myself, even if this does not get published, it will at least be helpful for my own work to have all of my art therapy directives more organized. For those of us who have had numerous art therapy jobs or work in hospitals or other settings where we see a variety of clients, this book may just be for you. I was fortunate to get my proposal selected for publishing and so began the writing and bad coffee sipping.

About This Book

As I began to shape this idea of a comprehensive guide where art therapy directives are organized and encompass the most common areas of treatment and diagnoses, I thought about who would use this book. I decided it would be a

DOI: 10.4324/9781003413363-1

reference style book (but not a boring one!) for new and seasoned art therapists as well as other trained mental health professionals to look up client-specific quick-at-a-glance session directives to guide their work with groups or individuals. Readers should be able to search by the population they are working with or the client's particular goal for their session such as grief work with children. Additionally, the reader can search the index by specific art medium, such as fiber art or watercolor, if they have a client who wants to work with a particular material. I hope this format was as successful in its straightforward nature as I intended it to be. With all that said, I am a Board Certified Art Therapist with a master's degree in art therapy and second master's degree in education. I am not a medical professional and do not assert to be one. I have given suggestions on art therapy directives that I have used and found effective in my previous experience. Please use your own best judgment as a trained mental health professional with this book for support and guidance. If you or a professional you are working with have concerns, seek medical advice. In my experience, working in acute care, the team approach is always the best. At certain times, a patient or client may need medical attention and traditional pharmaceutical prescriptions with the support of the therapist or art therapist.

History of Art Therapy

Next, I would like to give some background on the development of the field of art therapy and what exactly *is* an art therapy directive. Despite art therapy having roots in Freudian and Jungian psychoanalysis, it is a relatively young field of study. The first tracings of art therapy work were in the 1940s by the "mother of art therapy," Margaret Naumburg, when she began publishing her cases and titled them "dynamically oriented art therapy." "In 1940 Naumburg was the first to define art therapy as a separate mental health discipline and as a different form of psychotherapy." A second pioneer in the field, Edith Kramer, evolved around the same time. "Unlike Naumburg, Kramer argues that art therapists are not psychotherapists, and should not need to be. Her work relied very little, if any, on talking where as Naumburg, through verbal inquiry, intends to further the patient's conscious exploration of unconscious" (Borowski Junge, 2015). Other important pioneers and leaders in our field evolved from there including: Elinor Ulman, Judith Rubin, and Florence Cane. My gratitude to these strong and creative women leaders.

Some people have only heard of the term art therapy and do not really know what it is or is not. To begin, the broader field is called Creative Arts Therapy or Expressive Arts. Under those umbrella terms come the modalities, which include: (visual) art therapy, music therapy, dance/movement therapy, drama therapy, and expressive writing. This brings me to the fact that there are a number of myths about the field of art therapy that I would like to debunk. The most common myth is that art therapy is only for talented artists and creative people.

This could not be farther from the truth! In fact, I love to work with people who are intimidated by art the most. I mean, I really enjoy all my clients, but this is a special area of interest. Art therapy is about the process of art making not the end product. If clients are struggling with the art media rather than the topic at hand, I know I must have done something wrong. I generally pick art therapy mediums and directives that are easily attainable, where the client or patient can then focus more on their thoughts and feelings during the session rather than the art-making technique. I also want the art therapy project to be attainable; the last thing I would want is for the client to feel frustrated or disappointed in their own abilities. Unless for some reason the goal is to practice "messing up" which is also valid at times. So hopefully now you are convinced that anyone can participate in art therapy. Another common myth is that art therapy is only for children. While art therapy is a useful tool for children, it is most certainly not only for them. When we are young, our play is our work. We wake up and color or build, have a snack, use some sidewalk chalk, nap, dinner, maybe some more drawing before bed, and call it a day. Those were the days! Then as we progress to elementary and middle school we likely have art weekly and then somehow by high school, it becomes an elective. Yet we continue math and foreign languages throughout. Why do we lose our obligation to creativity as we get older? This is because it is not a fundamental part of our education like other subjects. So how could we expect adults to feel comfortable and competent in making art?! I believe this is where the intimidation about art comes from. Another important myth to discredit is that art therapists will analyze your art. Often, I have had people ask me, "what does my art mean?" I usually respond with "whatever it means to you." Art therapists are not psychics and will not analyze your artwork. Your artwork comes from you and you are the best at describing its purpose and meaning. Hopefully, this section has alleviated any reluctance about art therapy.

Art Therapy Today and Cultural Considerations

Next, I would like to discuss how arttherapy has progressed over time. The field of art therapy has evolved and grown since its inception in the 1940s. It was developed by intelligent, strong, creative women pioneers to whom I am proud to connect my professional lineage. With that said, the field of art therapy is predominantly facilitated by white, cisgender, straight women. I see this lack of diversity slowly beginning to shift, and it is something I am hopeful about. Just as our client populations are highly diverse, so should be the art therapists that are employed to work with them. It was not until 2019 that the American Art Therapy Association (AATA), the professional organization for art therapists, created a diversity, equity, and inclusion statement along with a planning group and strategic goals. "AATA critically examines our structures, values, and actions to ensure the continuous integration of diversity, equity, and inclusion within the organization and the art therapy community" (American Art Therapy

Association, 2019). I think it is important to consider why this may be. Beginning with training, the high cost of graduate school with minimal financial resources as well as below-average salaries for working art therapists are a problem within our field. The varied graduate programs within the fields of STEM provide graduate school assistance and research grants that are simply not available in the arts. Most art therapists will come out of graduate school with high debt into a profession of mostly work opportunities in the nonprofit or state-run sectors, which mainly offer inadequate compensations.

I would like to address how this lack of diversity may affect our clients and patients. One of the most significant barriers to access in art therapy would be the lack of centralized licensure in our field. Currently, we have a national credential, but this does not encompass state-by-state licensing regulations. In the state of New York, where I went to graduate school, for example, there is a License for Creative Arts Therapists however when my family and I moved to Virginia this particular license did not transfer. This can make it not only confusing for clients but also unattainable for art therapists. Without state licensing, art therapists cannot bill for services using health insurance and only charge out of pocket, which most people cannot afford. Another barrier to access for clients and patients would be access and cost of art materials. It is important for art therapists to consider how their practices, art therapy studios, or other workspaces may be intimidating or unintentionally unwelcoming to all. As art therapists, especially after the COVID-19 pandemic, we like to consider that we should be able to work with the simplest of materials. Therefore, it is important to consider the cost of various materials and the fact that most clientele may not have had access to or experience with these mediums, which can be off-putting. Additionally, it is important to consider cultural appropriation in art therapy directives. Mandalas are a staple in art therapy as well as many other culturally diverse techniques, some of which I even share in this book. It is critical when facilitating these types of techniques that we use the proper historically appropriate language, provide background and education on these techniques as well as pay homage to their cultural roots. Lastly, it is important to utilize the most up-to-date language to promote inclusion in our art therapy practices and utilize training and continuing education resources if not. Exploring our own implicit bias through self-exploration is vital in creating safe, affirming, and diverse spaces for our clients and patients. I have done my best to use the most up-to-date and inclusive language in this book, but will also continue to explore my own practice and commitment to expanding cultural diversity within the field of art therapy.

Art Therapy Directives

Next, I would like to explore what the title of this book means by defining the term art therapy directives. As mentioned above, the field of art therapy has varied techniques based on the history and pioneers in the field. Some styles may be more similar to Edith Kramer's, where there is little intervention or guidance from the art therapist. Many art therapy groups and sessions may be more "open studio" style in which the client is completely self-directed and uses any mediums they choose in front of them with little guidance from the art therapist. In this style, the art making takes the lead. While other art therapy frameworks provide more guidance for clients and patients. I prefer somewhat of a blended style and in-the-moment combination of creative process and art therapy techniques and guidance. It is in this instance that art therapists may have a "tool kit" of art therapy directives to utilize as needed, which are applicable based on the client's needs. Some other mental health professionals may ask what exactly an art therapy directive is? In facilitating individual, family, or group sessions, art therapists often use directives (or interventions) in their work to help clients explore a particular concern and use of specific art media. Art therapy directives are guidance or directions for creating art and often require use of specific art media, both of which are tailored to the client's particular need or goal for the session. Art therapists are often looking for new directives or to build a collection of them to have available as practitioners to refer to for various client needs. This is where I hope this book can serve my art therapy community. The art therapy community is one that I am proud to call myself part of and I would like to thank the pioneers, my predecessors, and mentors, especially for those whom I have acknowledged in the below art therapy directives and exercises.

Whom This Book Is Intended for

I intended this book to be used by trained art therapists and other mental health professionals as I mentioned. I also think this could be a useful resource for art therapeutic students as they are learning clinical experience and art therapeutic theories. However, I feel it is important to note that it is not a one-size-fits-all template to be followed exactly. Students learning about which mediums and applications are appropriate for which client takes time and experience, but I do hope it is informative and can inspire art therapy students to use their knowledge and gut instincts to drive their work. The beauty of gaining skills as an art therapist is having the ability to be very present with our clients and assess their needs as the session evolves.

Next, I would like to address an uncomfortable issue within the field of art therapy, and I might assume in other professions as well as it relates to this subject. This is the idea of "gatekeeping" our training secrets. Even some of the feedback I received on my peer review edits mentioned concern around the idea that we are minimizing our training by siphoning it down into a listing of art therapy directives. However, this is not my intention at all, but rather to bring awareness about our field to others that gatekeeping has potentially held us back from. For other mental health professionals who are using this book, I would like to give a background on art therapy training that some may not be aware of. To become a Registered Art Therapist, which is an entry-level clinician, a student must complete a master's degree in art therapy from an accredited program, which entails both coursework and practicum hours. Once the master's degree is attained, at least 1,000 additional post-education direct client contact hours of art therapy must also be completed plus an additional 100 hours of clinical supervision by an art therapist (Art Therapy Credentials Board, 2023). Through this art therapist can also gain board certification status through a national examination. With that said, art therapists and perhaps other trained mental health professionals need to work within their scope of practice. Just as an art therapist may integrate cognitive-behavioral techniques or specific trauma-related techniques into our work, perhaps the opposite could be done. In fact, I know it is done, so hopefully this will provide some guidance. However, the main goal of this book is to be a reminder of various art therapy directives and their application with the knowledge that as trained professionals we shift and adapt to what our client needs not using this book as an exacting template.

How to Use This Book

My goal with this book was to be a quick-at-a-glance reference style book, comprehensive, and organized resource for art therapists and other trained mental health professionals. Art therapists and other practitioners should be able to search by population, themes, and art media to find just the right project for their session, whether working with individuals, families, or groups. The chapters are simply organized in alphabetical order as to make it straightforward for the clinician. I have tried to encompass the majority of populations, diagnoses, and/ or goals in the chapter topics but know of course this may not be an exhaustive list. I also wanted art therapists to be able to use the index to search by art medium as an alternative means for finding art therapy directives based on media rather than topic. I have tried to include as much variety of media as possible in this book. I have included the following two-dimensional mediums: drawing with pencil, colored pencil, crayons, markers, charcoal, oil pastels, chalk pastels, and collage. I have included painting with watercolor pencils, watercolor paints, and acrylic. Three dimensionally I have included sculpting with various types of clay, plaster, and paper sculptures. In terms of fiber arts, I have projects using: knitting, crocheting, embroidery, and quilting. I have also included more nuanced media such as: digital arts, mosaic tiles, jewelry making, and materials from nature. However, the majority of the art therapy exercises will utilize basic two-dimensional materials. Of course, as trained art therapists, the medium can always be substituted to suit and adapt to the particular session or as requested by the client. Lastly, you will also notice that some of the art therapy directives have a web site link that would explain a specific technique through a video. I made these videos when the COVID-19 pandemic just began and the William & Mary Wellness Center quickly shifted to an online video format for art therapy and other wellness sessions. These videos encompass particular art therapy techniques that may be easier to follow through video rather than written instruction. My goal overall was to make this a simple well-organized book of art therapy interventions that are in one location rather than in various different books or online resources, and I hope for it to be helpful in that way.

Another important bit I would like to share about how to use this book has to do with the writing up of the art therapy directives. I have given brief overviews of each of the art therapy directives that give the main idea for a session in summary. As a trained art therapist or other mental health clinician, of course, you will have your own structure for groups or individual sessions. The way I structure an individual, family, or group session is based on the importance of a marked beginning, middle, and end. In general, I begin with a check-in with the client and generally introduce and discuss our main topic or goal for the session. Then there is a significant amount of time for art making and talking. Lastly, and most importantly, there is a time set aside for sharing and processing of the artwork. I have not necessarily described in each chapter or directive specific issues that should be discussed as art therapy professionals because we are well equipped to handle this individually and the moment which is where the power of the session lies.

Scope of Practice

This brings me to another important issue within the field of art therapy, which is scope of practice and I briefly touched on this above. This is the idea of art as therapy versus art therapy. As I mentioned above, I assume that other trained mental health professionals, not just art therapists, will utilize this book. Only registered art therapists can technically call themselves art therapists. It is important to note that there is a difference between art as therapy and art therapy as a practice. Art as therapy as an example would be a client using a coloring book and noticing that it is relaxing. Art therapy, however, is facilitated by a master's level registered art therapist. While the act of art making itself can feel "therapeutic" in that it is relaxing, promotes mindfulness, and has been proven to reduce blood pressure, it is not art therapy. Authentic art therapy is when a trained art therapist works with an individual, family, or group utilizing the creative process and psychological theories to improve mental health. I would also like to suggest that if you are not trained as an art therapist or are new to the field that you may want to try these art therapy directives on your own before facilitating them with a client. Not only would this be helpful from a technique standpoint but also more importantly it would help the therapist to understand what it would feel like to make this art piece and to feel the feelings that it may impart on the client. This might help the clinician be more prepared for the client's feelings and responses to the art in the session. Just as many of us in the mental health profession were recommended to work on ourselves in therapy as we progressed through our graduate programs, this would be a similarly beneficial training experience on a smaller scale level.

Theoretical Frameworks and Styles

Within the field of art therapy there are a number of different styles or frameworks from which a clinician could approach working with their clients, patients, families, and/or groups. Art therapy styles can include: person-centered, psychodynamic, assessment-based, Jungian, Gestalt, humanistic, mindfulness-based, psychoanalytic, positive, and transpersonal. Additionally, art therapists may integrate cognitive behavioral, dialectical behavioral, family systems, emotion-focused, play therapy, dance movement or yoga therapy, music therapy, or other types of modalities into their work. Lastly, the Expressive Therapies Continuum is an important framework from which many art therapists now consider it to be the predominant theory from which many art therapy sessions are conducted. It was developed and first written about in 1978 by art therapists Sandra Kagin and Vija Lusebrink in their seminal article "The Expressive Therapies Continuum" published in the journal *Art Psychotherapy*. The Expressive Therapies Continuum "is a conceptual model designed for, and of use to, the various fields of the art and expressive psychotherapies. The continuum is composed of four levels, representing four modes of interaction with the media theoretically assumed to reflect the different modes of human expression" (Kagin & Lusebrink, 1978). With the Expressive Therapies Continuum as the framework for client choice on materials, art therapists can utilize this book as a means to select or offer materials or suggest meaningful directives to clients within this context as well.

Even with all of the numerous options we have as art therapists for various mediums, counseling styles, theoretical frameworks, or art therapy directives I suggest in this book, we must still, as trained art therapists, use our in-the-moment tools that best suit each client. Please know that this book is not meant to be used as an instruction manual but more of a listing of options for the art therapist to refer to. It is not to suggest that all clients with a certain diagnosis or session goal must use just the prescribed art therapy directive. Many of the art therapy directives I wrote about could overlap or be utilized in several of the chapters. It is my hope that the art therapist can alter or adapt any of these as needed. Likewise, another important note I would like to make about this book is that it is not my intention to pathologize or categorize clients and patients into diagnostic "boxes." Humans are complicated and one size does not fit all. Therefore, please know that I understand and empathize with the impact of a diagnosis or other mental health struggle and am in awe of my clients and patients who have courageously opened up and attended art therapy or other treatment forms.

Recommended Readings

Lastly, you will notice in some chapters and sections that I have recommended related readings. Please note that I have not received anything for these recommendations just that I have found them relevant and useful for a deeper dive into certain topics. In some circumstances, I have only read a portion of the book, while in other books, I have read over and over. I am thankful to the fellow art therapists, psychologists, and authors for sharing their knowledge, which, in some cases, is very specific and contains years of expertise.

Reference List

American Art Therapy Association. (2019). *AATA Board of Directors Approves Diversity, Equity, and Inclusion Vision Statement.* Retrieved from https://arttherapy.org/news-aata-dei-vision-statement/#:~:text=During%20the%20April%202019%20in-person%20board%20meeting%2C%20the,within%20the%20organization%20and%20the%20art%20therapy%20community.

Art Therapy Credentials Board. (2023). *About the Credentials.* Retrieved from https://atcb.org/about-the-credentials/.

Borowski Junge, M. (2015). History of art therapy. In T. D. E. Gussak & M. L. Rosal (Eds.), *The Wiley handbook of art therapy (Wiley clinical psychology handbooks)* (1st Edition, pp. 7–16). Hoboken, NJ: John Wiley & Sons. doi: 10.1002/9781118306543.ch1.

Kagin, S., & Lusebrink, V. (1978). The expressive therapies continuum. *Art Psychotherapy, 5*(4), 171–180. doi: 10.1002/9781118306543.

Chapter 2

Adolescents and Young Adults

I worked on the adolescent unit of a large psychiatric hospital in Vermont for a number of years, and often when I told people this, they would shudder. You have to like teenagers to work with them. There were staff that would come and go, and I would find my co-workers who had the hardest time working with the teens also had really difficult adolescence themselves. Although those years are a challenging time for even the best of us! One thing I always noticed at the various psychiatric hospitals I worked at was how the staff would often mirror the patients on their particular unit. I found this also included the unit's general physical environment as well. The adolescent unit, where I felt embarrassingly comfortable, was significantly messier and more disorganized than other units, similar to my own teenager's current bedroom. The staff, whom I loved, were likewise silly, messy, and high energy, which worked well with the clientele. One continuing education training I attended facetiously described all teenagers as exhibiting Borderline Personality Disorder traits. This makes a lot of sense. Developmentally, adolescents are torn between still wanting their parent's comfort and safety with a burgeoning need for independence. Therefore, art therapy directives designed for teenagers must contain this balance as well, just enough structure and guidance paired with a lot of creative freedom.

Description: Comic Panel

Supplies: Comic Panel Printouts or Drawing Paper, Pencil, Ruler, Eraser, Colored Pencil, and Fine Point Markers

Directions: I usually have a few blank pre-made comic panels in my supply closet on hand and have noticed its mostly adolescents who are drawn to these. Since comic strips tell a full story rather than a single image, I find this exercise in particular lends itself to any sort of narrative your adolescent client may need to work through. Alternatively, the comic strip could be about a meta character for the client. Also its important to note, many clients enjoy the process of making the entire comic including the comic panels rather than use the comic template.

DOI: 10.4324/9781003413363-2

Description: Digital Art Altered Self-Portrait

Supplies: Camera or Smart Phone, Computer or Tablet, Digital Art Applications, Photocopy Machine, Printer, Photocopy of a Portrait, Scissors, Glue Stick, and Cardstock Paper

Directions: Adolescents are adept at and drawn to digital media and therefore projects using this medium are one way to drawn them in. There are several ways to create an abstract or an altered self-portrait using various computer programs, the most well-known being Adobe Photoshop®.

Variation: However if computers are not available, a similar alternative could be to manipulate photo copies of portrait photos using collage or other image transfer techniques. I personally have enjoyed using Citra-Solv in this way. For specific Citra Solv image transfer instructions see the section below. However for a collage technique, begin with a photocopy of a portrait photo. This could be cut up and manipulated and then glued back down onto a piece of cardstock paper creating a new altered self-portrait.

Further Reading: For more in-depth work on digital art and art therapy, I suggest *The Handbook of Art Therapy and Digital Technology* edited by Cathy Malchiodi (2018).

Description: Photo Transfer

Supplies: Photocopy of a Photograph, Canvas Board, Citra-Solv®, Cotton Balls, Paper Towels, and a Metal Spoon

Directions: Being that adolescents and young adults are in a foremost state of transition in their lifespans, the process of photo transfer is fitting. This is a simple technique that requires minimal chemicals especially since Citra-Solv® is made from plant based, non toxic materials. Ask the client to bring in an important photo or perhaps something specific to the work you are doing together. Then make a photocopy of the photo using a toner based machine or print from the computer. Be sure to open windows because the Citra-Solv® has a strong aroma, despite being non toxic. Place the photo copy down onto the canvas board and apply dabs of the Citra-Solv® to the back of the photocopy with cotton balls making sure it gets completely covered, but is not runny. Then use the back of a metal spoon to burnish the print onto the canvas board, but be careful to not tear the paper. Then gently peel the photo copy paper off the canvas board. I always warn clients that often photo transfers look slightly different or manipulated which is the beauty in them. This is also a magnificent and important metaphor at this developmental stage that being slightly different can be wonderful.

Contraindicated: Some people have a stronger sensitivity to smell, and the use of Citra-Solv® would not be recommended due to its intense citrus aroma.

Description: Secret Word Mandala

Supplies: Drawing Paper Cut into Large Circles, Pencil, Eraser, Colored Pencil, and Fine Point Markers

Directions: Ask clients to think of a word that is meaningful to them or relates to the focus of their therapeutic work. Begin by having clients fold their circle into eighths. Starting with it folded into a one-eighth sized section, ask the clients write their word using block letters filling the triangle section completely. It is important to start with a pencil and eraser because there will be some adjusting along the way. Then open the folds, making it back into a full circle and repeat this on the other seven sections. Once this word has been written eight times around, use eraser and pencil to connect the letters in each section to one another (see example). Once the word is connected in

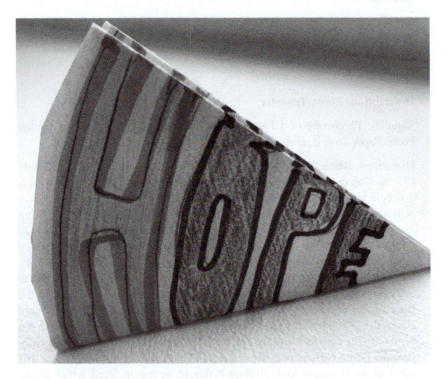

Figure 2.1 Secret Word Mandala (Folded).
Source: Photograph and artwork by the author.

all the eight sections, clients can go over it with fine point permanent marker and add color to their liking. This will begin to look more like an abstract mandala rather than the word as it develops. When clients share their artwork at the conclusion of the group, each client can then go into more depth about the meaning behind their significant word.

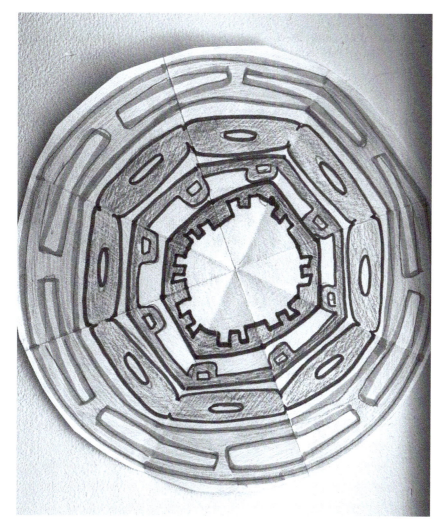

Figure 2.2 Secret Word Mandala (Completed).

Source: Photograph and artwork by the author.

Contra-Indication: This is a more advanced drawing and fine motor exercise and would be contra indicated for clients who have trouble working with small details or have trouble concentrating for an extended period of time.

Variation: Based on what the client is working on the focus of this directive can easily be adapted. For example, the client's word could relate to their self-esteem, recovery, personality etc.

Reference List

Malchiodi, C. (Ed.). (2018). *The handbook of art therapy and digital technology*. London: Jessica Kingsley Publishers.

Chapter 3

Anger Management

Anger is one of the most common emotions clients may exhibit or want to work on in sessions. Some clients may be "assigned" to therapy because of their anger from their employer or other outside sources. People may struggle with anger due to past trauma, grief, job loss, addiction, illness, divorce, or other unfair life struggles. Many people are too quick to jump to anger, while others may be afraid to express it. Anger is often called a secondary emotion because it can be a way to cover up other more vulnerable feelings. In general, the use of clay can be helpful in working on anger because of its physical nature. Sholt and Gavron (2006) confirm that "the many opportunities of modeling in clay furnish countless ways in which anger can be expressed or ventilated, such as scratching, clasping, stabbing, throwing, smashing, and so on. As mentioned above, these emotional expressions are made through the most primal and procedural mode of communication, through tactile contact and on a somatic level." One psychiatric hospital I worked at had a clay wheel for patients to use, which was a unique and special piece of art equipment for a hospital setting that was generously donated. The wedging, pushing, and pulling involved in preparing the clay can be a release, while the centering on the wheel can be calming and meditative in nature. Hand building with clay is beneficial on its own, but if there is access to a clay wheel this can provide a second layer where a calm meditative state can also be accessed. Below are a few art therapy exercises to help sublimate anger using a variety of mediums.

Description: Anger Container

Supplies: Air Dry Clay or Traditional, Ceramic Clay (if a kiln is available), Water Cup, and Clay Tools

Directions: Clients will begin by wedging the clay to remove air bubbles and warm it up. This physical act can be settling and a healthy example to clients on how to transform aggressive feelings into something more productive. Clients can then create any vessel shape or type of bowl which can symbolize a container for their anger. Clients could also possibly etch words, phrases or symbols into the clay that relate to their work on anger.

DOI: 10.4324/9781003413363-3

Description: Anger Iceberg

Supplies: Drawing Paper, Pencil, Colored Pencils or Markers

Directions: Provide psycho education to clients about the Anger Iceberg Theory created by Drs. Julie and John Gottman. This means that often when people are angry there are a myriad of different emotions beneath the surface similar to that of an iceberg where the majority of the iceberg is beneath the waterline. I usually also show clients The Gottman Institute's handout on this as well (Gottman, 2023). Clients can then use colored pencil or other two-dimensional materials to draw their own anger iceberg incorporating words both above and below the surface specific to their personal experience.

Description: Breaking and Rebuilding

Supplies: Colored Paper, Cardboard, or other Scrap Materials, Oil Pastel, Marker, Scissors, Pipe Cleaners, Tissue Paper, Hot Glue or Glue Sticks

Directions: Clients can write words, names, or images on the paper that may trigger feelings of anger. Then clients are able to physically crumple up, cut, or tear up these pages which usually feels cathartic for most. Clients can then rebuild with these pieces and add additional materials such as pipe cleaners or tissue paper to turn this into a transformed sculptural piece. This is also a great exercise for groups where everyone can then make a collaborative sculpture from their individual torn pieces rebuilt together.

Variation: Similar in feeling but more of a unique medium would be working with mosaics. It does come with added safety issues though which is important to note. For this exercise, clients can break plates and rebuild as a mosaic to also internalize this concept of breaking and rebuilding. As a safety tip when I have done this exercise with groups in the past, I have found that placing the plates into a canvas bag before breaking them is helpful for safety and clean up.

Description: Stress Ball

Supplies: Latex Balloons, Flour, Funnel, and Permanent Markers

Directions: Provide psycho education to clients about the use of a tool like a stress ball for in times of need during anger or other distressing situations. Begin with a latex balloon and place the funnel inside the balloon. Next add flour to desired amount, getting air out when near completion. Lastly, tie a secure knot on top. If working with younger clients, they can draw and decorate the outside of the stress ball using colored permanent markers.

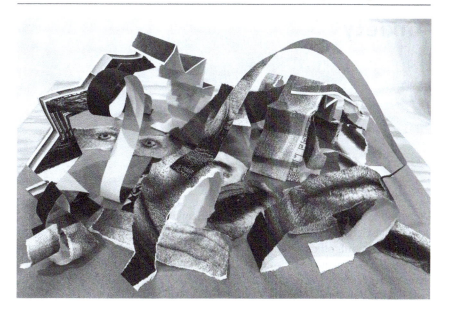

Figure 3.1 Collaborative Anger Sculpture.

Source: Photograph and artwork by the author.

Reference List

Gottmann Institute. (2023). *The Anger Iceberg*. Retrieved from https://www.gottman. com/blog/the-anger-iceberg/.

Sholt, M., & Gavron, T. (2006). Therapeutic qualities of clay-work in art therapy and psychotherapy: A review. *Art Therapy: Journal of the American Art Therapy Association*, *23*(2), 66–72. doi: 10.1080/07421656.2006.10129647.

Chapter 4

Anxiety

Perhaps one of the most frequent reasons a client may be seeking treatment is because of anxiety. Anxiety is common and can be situational, persistent, or often co-occurring with other diagnoses. Within the broader field of the creative arts therapies, movement-based and body-focused therapies such as dance movement therapy and yoga are really effective. Since anxiety can affect the body so profoundly with symptoms, such as increased heart rate, nausea, sweaty palms, etc., clients will find relief through some of these movement-based techniques. Although I am trained as a visual art therapist, my graduate program at Pratt Institute was paired with dance movement therapists. Despite my initial terror, this has been a valuable part of my training and work experience. I believe strongly in the integration of the various creative arts therapies when clinically appropriate. Personally, I have long used yoga as a tool for my own self-care and often incorporate techniques into my clinical work. I found it beneficial to get the 200-hour teacher training and/or attend continuing education trainings on the integration of these two fields. Below are various directives I have used in groups and with individuals that have helped reduce anxiety symptoms.

Description: Five Drawings

Supplies: 5 sheets of 8.5 x 11 Drawing Paper (or one larger sheet divided into sections), Pencil, Eraser, and a Simple Still Life (set up or photo of one)

Directions: This directive is derived from a traditional drawing technique that I adapted into a mindfulness based drawing exercise. Focusing intently on the present moment can help reduce anxiety by giving clients the ability to control where their own thoughts go. Present the clients with a simple image or still life that could be used to draw from. Give basic psycho education about mindfulness and non-judgmental stance before beginning. Clients will draw the still life five different times so therefore it is important to emphasize brief sketches, spending roughly 3–5 min on each. Sketch one – is a *blind drawing* of the still life, meaning they only look at the objects as they draw them, not the paper. Sketch two- is a *contiguous line drawing* of the still life,

DOI: 10.4324/9781003413363-4

meaning they must keep their pencil on the paper throughout. Sketch three – is drawing with the *non-dominant hand*. Sketch four – is drawing the image from *upside down* and for this is it helpful to take a photo and rotate it for the clients to draw. Sketch five – is a *traditional drawing* of the still life. It is interesting to compare all five drawings at the conclusion and also take note of how concentrating in the present moment can reduce anxiety.

Description: Lavender Eye Pillow

Supplies: Fabric, Scissors, Thread, Needles, Rice, Dried Lavender or Essential Oil

Directions: This directive is one that I learned at the Brattleboro Retreat from my skilled art therapy colleagues. Lavender is well known as a naturopathic technique to reduce anxiety symptoms. Clients begin by selecting fabric and cutting it into a rectangular shape; they will need two of these rectangles. Next sew (either by hand or by machine if available) the rectangles together on all but one of the short sides of the rectangle with the patterns facing inward. After this, the rectangle shape can be turned right side out. Using a paper funnel and teamwork, rice can be added to desired amount. The more rice the harder and heavier the eye pillow but less rice can yield a softer more malleable eye pillow. At this point, clients can add the dried lavender or drops of essential oil to their desired amount. Finally, the rectangular pillow can be sewn shut. To keep the seams internal, I usually fold the ends inward before sewing shut.

Variation: By altering the size, shape, and materials put inside, clients can also create more of a stress ball rather than an eye pillow.

Contraindicated: Sewing materials can be dangerous if safety is a concern, such as in certain hospital settings. Additionally, some people have a stronger sensitivity to smell, and the use of essential oils would not be recommended.

Description: Self-Soothing Fidget

Supplies: Various Types of Decorative Beads, Letter Beads, Cord, Scissors and Lobster Clasp

Directions: Begin the session with basic psycho education around coping skills for anxiety including positive self-talk, mindfulness, sensory tools, and distraction techniques. Have clients think of a self-soothing word for themselves in times of increased anxiety. Examples could include: peace, breathe, or slow down. Clients can then create a self-soothing fidget using cord and beads to spell out their specific word reminder. This also doubles as something to fidget with in their pocket or it can be attached to bags or other items to use as needed.

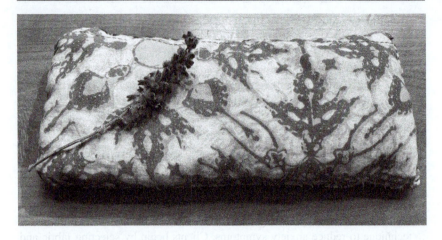

Figure 4.1 Lavender Eye Pillow.
Source: Photograph by the author.

Description: Yoga & Art Therapy

Supplies: Space Enough for Movement, Chalk Pastel, Oil Pastel, or Crayons

Directions: After considering contraindications and receiving consent from the client or group members, begin the session with three to five rounds of sun salutations. This can be performed seated or standing. Starting a session with movement can help clients feel more present and grounded utilizing "bottom up" versus "top down" therapeutic work. When ready, clients can create a piece using various mediums based on how this movement felt. I have found chalk pastels work well because of their free flowing quality. It can also be beneficial for clients to note their emotion state or anxiety level before and after the session as a tangible marker of how affective this could be for them in the future on their own.

Contraindicated: Yoga and body-based work is not recommended for those who have experienced trauma unless working with a highly trained dance movement therapist or yoga therapist as this can be triggering. Also, this would not be recommended for clients who are uncomfortable with their bodies for various reasons or have physical limitations or injuries.

Further Reading: For more in-depth work in this field, I suggest *Integrating Art Therapy and Yoga Therapy* by Karen Gibbons as well as the renowned *The Body Keeps the Score: Brain, Mind, and Body Healing of Trauma* by Bessel van der Kolk (Gibbons, 2015; Van der Kolk, 2015).

Reference List

Gibbons, K. (2015). *Integrating art therapy and yoga therapy*. London: Jessica Kingsley Publishers.
Van der Kolk, B. (2015). *The body keeps the score: Brain, mind, and body healing of trauma*. New York, NY: Penguin.

Chapter 5

Autism Spectrum Disorder

Sensory Integration techniques are a valuable tool when working with clients on the Autism Spectrum, which is why art therapy pairs well. These techniques and tools can include certain aromas in your space, various music or other sounds, calm or colorful lighting, and various tactile tools. Some of the most common tactile sensory tools are weighted blankets, putties, eye pillows, stress balls, and chewing toys. I was also fortunate enough to be trained by renowned occupational therapist Tina Champagne while I worked at an inpatient psychiatric hospital in Vermont. We collaborated on integrating sensory tools into the adolescent unit's milieu. The benefits of creating a space like this in a hospital setting were outstanding, as patients were able to access this room as needed throughout their hospital stay. It also proved to be a learning experience for gathering helpful tools for at home. More recently, I have had the privilege of working at the One Child Center for Autism in Williamsburg, Virginia, providing art therapy groups for neurodiverse children, adolescents, and their families on the community outreach level. Art therapy blends well with sensory integration techniques because of the many tactile and visual sensory mediums. A few mediums that I have noticed that are particularly useful for sensory-related projects are: modeling clay, acrylic and watercolor paint, and fiber arts. Below are a few art therapy directives that I have found particularly useful when working with neurodiverse clients and groups.

Further Reading: For an expert opinion with inventive techniques, I recommend the book *Special Interests in Art Therapy With Autistic People: A Neurodiversity-Positive Approach to Empower and Engage Participants* by Jessica Woolhiser Stallings (2022).

Description: Pillow Stuffed Animal Making

Supplies: Soft Fleece Fabric, Needles, Thread, Cotton Stuffing, Scissors, Fabric Markers, Buttons, Drawing Paper, Pen, and Essential Oils

Directions: For younger clients, making their own self-soothing item to have as a coping skill that they created themselves can be empowering. I have

DOI: 10.4324/9781003413363-5

had clients create simple stuffed animals from socks to more intricately sewn stuffed animals. For a more advanced pillow stuffed animal, I like to use soft fleece fabric. Next cut out the basic shape of the stuffed animal, which can be more abstract since it will also serve as a sort of pillow. Cut out two of these starter shapes. Using a needle and thread, sew the two pieces facing inward so that the seam will be internal. Leave a few inches open when sewing it shut. Turn the material so that it is facing outward and fill it with the stuffing. It can also be meaningful to put a special note inside with words of empowerment or whatever goal the client may be working on as an embodied reminder inside this transitional object. An added sensory tool could also be to put drops of essential oil on the stuffing before sewing up the pillow stuffed animal.

Contraindicated: Some people have a stronger sensitivity to smell, and the use of essential oils would not be recommended.

Description: Quilling

Supplies: Thin Strips of Colored Paper, Cardstock for Mounting, Pencil or Quilling Tool, Glue and/or Glue Stick

Directions: While not a traditional art therapy medium, the act of making tiny paper quills can be really satisfying for some. However for those who

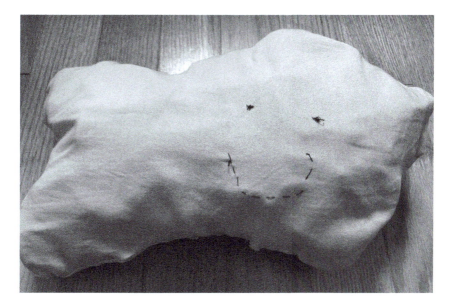

Figure 5.1 Pillow Stuffed Animal.

Source: Photograph by the author. Artwork by Drew Balascio.

enjoy tiny details and precision, quilling could be just the right medium. Paper quilling or some times referred to as 'filigree' is the art of rolling small strips of paper to form tightly wound coils that can be joined together to create an image. I encourage simplicity, perhaps beginning by making one uncomplicated image to start. While there is a specific quilling tool, I have had clients simply roll the paper between their fingers or wrap it around a pencil to start. Quills can be manipulated into various shapes by pressing on them and combined to create one larger image.

Contraindicated: This can be a challenging fine motor skill which could be helpful or frustrating based on the client.

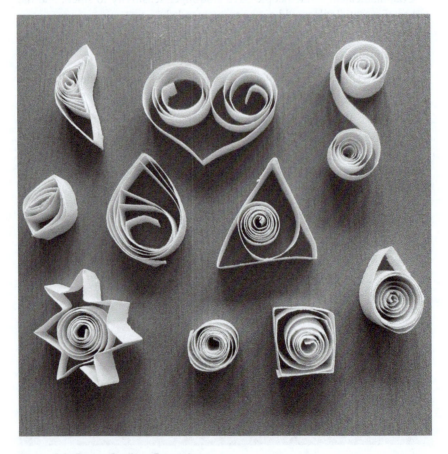

Figure 5.2 Paper Quilling Examples.

Source: Photograph by the author.

Description: Sensory Sculptures

Supplies: White Air Dry Clay (Model Magic® is my preference for this project), Washable Markers, Essential Oils, and Clay Tools

Directions: Clients can begin by warming up the clay in their hands or on the table in front of them. Clients can also add essential oils at this point as they work with the clay. Next have clients roll out the clay flat with a tool or often we just use the washable marker to do this. Next, they can give the clay color by drawing onto it with washable markers. Then they will mash it up again until the color blends completely. In order to gain a deep color this will need to be repeated a number of times, which in itself is a technique that some will enjoy. Once the desired color is reached, clients can shape it into any object they like. I also let clients know that if they enjoy using it more as a sensory tool it can be stored in an air tight container for a couple days but will eventually dry up if not.

Contraindicated: Sensory aversion can be an issue with clay or marker getting on client's hands. A helpful option could be to wear rubber gloves. Again, be advised of the sensitivity to smell for some with the use of essential oils.

Description: Sensory Tool Kit

Supplies: Large Cardboard Box or Shoe Box, Magazines, Scissors, Glue Sticks, Two-Dimensional Drawing Materials, Decoupage Glue and Brush (Mod Podge® is my preference for this project)

Directions: I learned about sensory integration tool kits when I was working on the adolescent unit an in-patient psychiatric hospital in Brattleboro, Vermont. As I mentioned above, we piloted a sensory integration initiative on our unit. I would usually begin this art therapy session by discussing with clients what their preferred sensory tools are. Some examples could include: putty, chewing gum, stress balls, or weighted lap pads. Next we create a decorative sensory box to keep these items in for times of need. Clients can collage or draw soothing images and colors to the outside of their tool kits as an added benefit. This is a personalized tool kit that the client can go to independently when they need to take a break and use their specific sensory tools.

Reference List

Woolhiser Stallings, J. (2022). *Special interests in art therapy with autistic people: A neurodiversity-positive approach to empower and engage participants*. London: Jessica Kingsley Publishers.

Chapter 6

Children

One of the biggest misconceptions about art therapy is that it is mainly for children. However, ironically, I have found working with younger children not as easy as one might think. In my experience, the best child art therapy directives need to be structured just enough for the child to feel safe but also for them to be excited about the art making process. A foundational education in children's natural developmental stages of art making is crucial. Since otherwise normative images could potentially be misinterpreted. Many parents or other traditional non-art therapist clinicians often ask "the meaning" of their children's drawings or the symbolism. While some images may be very direct and straightforward, I have found it dangerous to try and "interpret" children's drawings, even as trained art therapists. Children create many varied images that may look like one thing while they may mean something completely different. Talking about our client's artwork with them and their purpose is always the best way to learn about their personal experience. Safety of materials with younger children or in hospital settings is also another important factor for the art therapist to consider. Below are a few art therapy examples that I have found work well with children of varying abilities.

Further Reading: For more in-depth reading on art therapy with children, I suggest the preeminent book *Child Art Therapy* by Judith Rubin (2005).

Description: Dream Catchers

Supplies: Metal or Wooden Hoops, Embroidery Floss, Needles, Beads, Feathers, and Scissors

Directions: I begin this art therapy directive always by paying respect to and giving education around the Native American history of Dream Catchers. The reason I find this project meaningful with children is that often fears, or anxiety come out through their bedtime and sleep (or lack of). I have found that while children are working collaboratively with a therapist on this project significant details are shared about worries or concerns that the client

DOI: 10.4324/9781003413363-6

may have. Clients begin by picking their desired materials with varying color choices for embroidery floss, feathers, and beads. I usually have clients start by attaching the string with a knot to the hoop. Clients can add beads to the string as they go and wrap the string in various locations of the hoop, making it as symmetrical or simple as they prefer. Additionally, clients can tie a string from the base of the loop and add dangling beads and feathers. Lastly, add a string with a loop to hang the completed Dream Catcher.

Description: Future Self-Portrait

Supplies: Watercolor, Tempera, or Acrylic Paint, Paint Palette, Paint Brushes, Water Cup, Paper Towel, Canvas or Watercolor Paper

Directions: Ask the client to think of what they would like their life and world to be like when they get older. Clients can use any type of paint to create a vision of themselves as an older person or adult. Around the outside of the self-portrait the client can put items to represent their interests, career, family or other lifestyle changes they would like to have in their life when they are older.

Description: Home

Supplies: Drawing Paper, Scissors, Pencil, Eraser, Crayons, Colored Pencils, Markers or Pastels

Directions: Ask clients to create a drawing of their house and its surroundings. If the client is between two homes, they can create two different versions, one at a time. Next, have the client put all their loved ones, family members, pets, and extended family members in the picture. In order to get to know the client more, I would suggest a less-is-more approach with regard to giving direction. As an art therapist, I stay away from any type of analysis, especially with children, since their drawings can look very different from what they may have intended. Generally, I ask the client to tell me what's in their drawing and why they included it. It should come from the client not the art therapist.

Variation: For much younger clients, a pre-made template of a house can be a helpful boundary for their drawing.

Note: This is a different art therapy directive than the traditional House-Tree-Person art therapy assessment.

Description: Power Word

Supplies: Jewelry String, Clasps, Scissors, Various Beads, and Letter Beads

Directions: The main focus of this directive can be tailored to the specific work with the client, but for this exercise we will focus on empowerment.

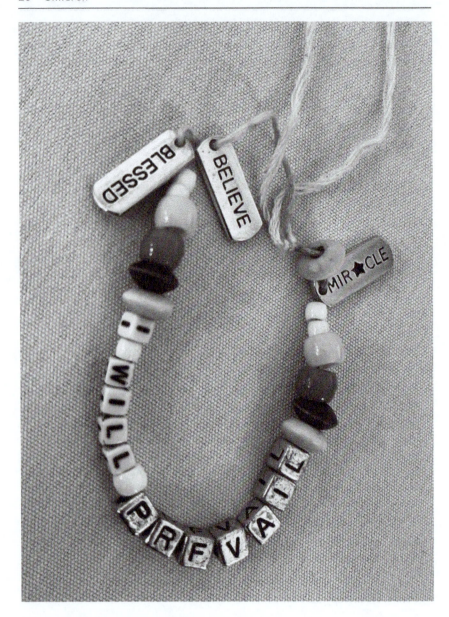

Figure 6.1 Power Word Jewelry.

Source: Photograph and artwork by Raven Pierce.

Ask the client to think of a word that gives them power or builds their self-esteem. Clients can work with various decorative beads and lettered beads to spell their particular empowering word or phrase (i.e., strength, persevere, "you got this!"). Using various types of jewelry making clasps this could be attached to a backpack, water bottle, worn as a bracelet or anywhere else noticeable for the child to have around them as a reminder.

Reference List

Rubin, J. (2005). *Child Art Therapy*. Hoboken, NJ: John Wiley & Sons.

Chapter 7

Depression

Many art therapy directives focus on calming, self-expression, or introspection. The biggest challenge when working with clients experiencing depression is the opposite, drawing up of energy. Depression can be situational, acute, prolonged, and/or cyclical. In my work at in-patient hospitals, it is one of the most common reasons for treatment. Often, clients will retreat to their rooms or may miss appointments if working outpatient with an art therapist. The hopeful goal of an art therapy directive when working with clients suffering from depression is to meet them where they are at, but with the goal of an increase of vitality by the end of the session. With art therapy, a sense of accomplishment is an added benefit when clients are able to leave with an actual physical reminder of their hard work in the session. Anecdotally, as art therapists, we can share how art therapy has benefited our patients and clients struggling with depression, but Thyme et al. (2007) conducted a study that confirms it. They looked at women with depression. Half of the group received traditional verbal therapy, while the second half received art therapy. The results of the study showed that art therapy was a valuable treatment for women with depression. Below are some art therapy directives that could be effective for working with client's varying degrees of depression.

Description: Act the Opposite

Supplies: Mixed Media Paper, Colored Pencil, Marker, Watercolor Pencil, or Pastels

Directions: Discuss with the client depressive behaviors they have been engaging in; for example: isolating, skipping groups or classes, sleeping too much. Provide psycho education around the Dialectical Behavior Therapy technique called "Opposite Action." Ask clients to select one of the behaviors that has been most prevalent for them and then have them consider an opposite behavior. Clients may need guidance brainstorming opposing behaviors. They can use any type of two-dimensional materials to depict this opposite

DOI: 10.4324/9781003413363-7

action or possibly a few of them. An example could be if the client has been isolating, they could create an image of themselves at the movies with some friends. One of the beautiful elements of art therapy is this ability to "practice" through the art making, as in this case it can serve as a warm up for actually completing these activities.

Description: Gratitude Tree

Supplies: Water Color Paper, Watercolor Pencils or Markers, Watercolor Paints, Watercolor Brushes Water Cup, Paper Towels, and Fine Point Permanent Markers for Writing

Directions: Negativity is a common and stubborn symptom of depression. In this directive, clients are asked to think instead about things small and big in their life they are grateful for. Clients can use any two dimensional medium to create a tree on their paper as the base. However for blending I have recommended watercolor as a medium of choice for this project. While not necessary to explain to the client, but often the tree is the symbol for the self in art therapy. Ask clients to think of anything in their life they are grateful for. Depending on the severity of their depressive symptoms, this could be something very minor (a favorite food) to something more profound (a second chance in life). At this point, the client can write as many of these things as they can think of anywhere on the tree, perhaps as leaves or engraved into the bark.

Description: HopeFULL

Supplies: Colored Paper, Scissors, Colored Pencils, Pencil, Eraser, and Clear Plastic Ball Ornaments

Directions: One of the benchmark symptoms of depression is hopelessness. For this art therapy directive, work with the client to think about things they might actually be hopeful about. Depending on the severity of the client's depression, this may be challenging. This can include a very small thing like- watching a favorite television show later in the day or bigger perspective item like starting therapy. For this art therapy directive, the client will need a clear plastic ball ornament. These can be purchased online or at any craft supply stores. Starting in the session, ask the client to try and think of one thing they are hopeful about and write it on a small strip of colored paper. Place this inside the ornament; they generally open and close on a center seam. Ask the client to try and think of one per day or one per week, whatever amount you feel is doable for the client. As the ornament gets filled with small strips of colored paper, it can not only look beautiful but be a visual reminder to the client of all the things they are hopeful about in their life.

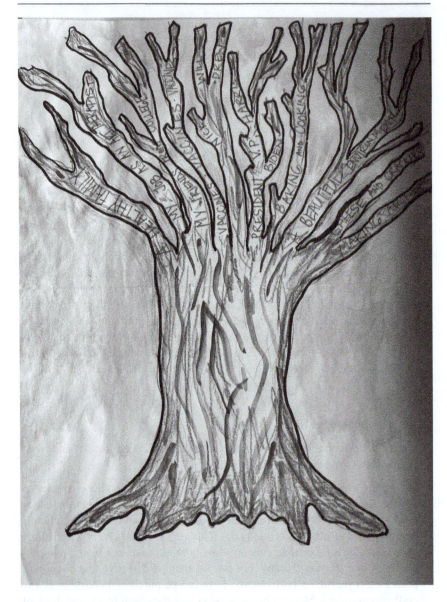

Figure 7.1 Gratitude Tree Watercolor.

Source: Photograph and artwork by the author.

Description: Portrait by the Art Therapist

Supplies: Mixed Media Paper, Pencil, Eraser, Pastels, Watercolor Paints or Acrylic Paint, Paint Palette, Paint Brushes, Water Cup, and Paper Towels

Directions: One of my internships during my graduate degree in art therapy was at an in-patient mental health unit inside a hospital in north western Massachusetts. My art therapy supervisor Merry was kind, gentle, and skilled. Often patients were too acutely depressed to participate in art therapy group. A couple of times I was lucky enough to witnessed her draw a portrait of the patient when they were unable to take part in a traditional way. She would talk with them and take in every detail of their being through her portraiture. This gives patients the feeling of being seen and engaging with even when they may feel invisible or hopeless.

Reference List

Thyme, K. E., Sundin, E. C., Gustaf, S., Lindstrom, B., Eklof, H., & Wiberg, B. (2007). The outcome of short-term psychodynamic art therapy compared to short-term psychodynamic verbal therapy for depressed women. *Psychoanalytic Psychotherapy, 21*(3), 250–264. doi: 10.1016/j.aip.2017.10.003.

Chapter 8

Eating Disorders

In my work at eating disorder treatment centers, it was the anxiety and rumination that struck me the most with the patients I worked with. I noticed that mediums such as knitting or crocheting were very helpful in keeping nervous hands busy. The benefit of knitting and crocheting is that once the technique is acquired, patients could knit or crochet in groups or while talking with their providers. Therefore, broadly speaking, knitting and crocheting is a helpful medium for those affected by eating disorders. Another common theme that many people with eating disorders struggle with is perfectionism. This can unfortunately become a focus of art making, consequently projects that are more abstract and don't have to be realistic are essential. The beautiful thing about art making that can be helpful to eating disorder patients is the indirect nature of our work. Any art therapist who has worked in a treatment center for eating disorders will notice the silence, it can be very challenging to get patients to talk and this is where the art can lead. Below are a few art therapy directives that may be useful for work clients struggling with an eating disorder.

Further Reading: For more in-depth work in this field, I suggest the book *Drawing From Within: Using Art to Treat Eating Disorders* by Lisa Hinz (2006).

Description: Create a Placemat

Supplies: Photos of Important People or Pets, Collage Magazine and Paper Scraps, Scissors, Glue Sticks, and Laminating Equipment

Directions: Mealtime in a treatment center or at home is one of the most challenging times when in recovery. Patients can create a collage placemat using photos of friends, loved ones, pets to help comfort them during meals. Patients could also include inspirational quotes, words, or motivational images as well. The art therapist may want to laminate the collages for preservation and use during numerous meals.

DOI: 10.4324/9781003413363-8

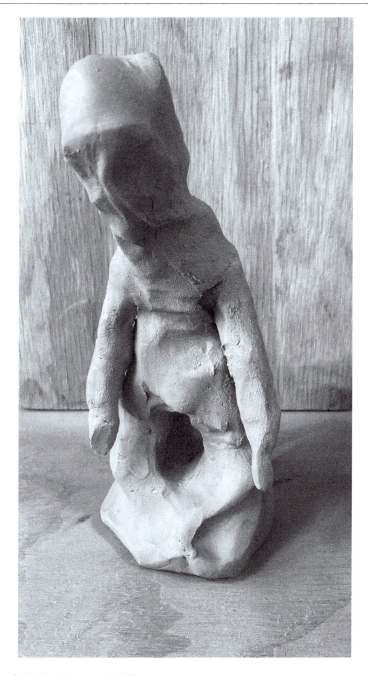

Figure 8.1 Clay Image of "Ed".

Source: Photograph and artwork by the author.

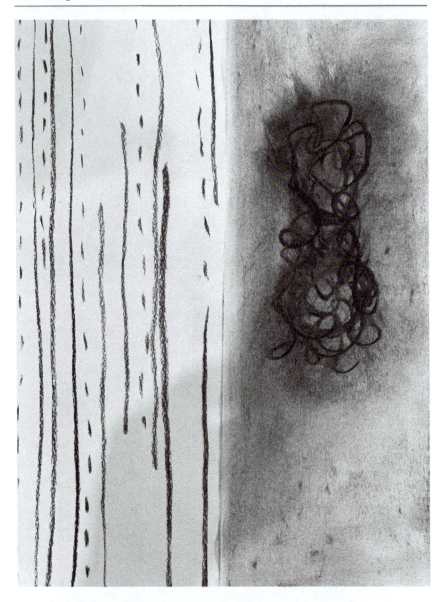

Figure 8.2 Charcoal Drawing of Recovery Dialectics: *Fear of Change and Wanting to Recover.*

Description: Drawing "Ed"

Supplies: Air Dry Clay, Water Cup, Clay Tools, Drawing Paper, Pencil, Eraser, Markers, and Colored Pencils

Directions: Patients in recovery often use the name "Ed" to refer to the negative voice or thoughts related to their eating disorder behaviors. In this directive, patients are asked to give an image or abstract being form to "Ed." This is useful because it can create separation between the patient and their eating disorder rather than being part of who they are as a person.

Description: Knit Blanket

Supplies: Yarn, Scissors, Knitting Needles or Knitting Loom

Directions: As I mentioned in the chapter introduction, knitting is a beneficial medium for those receiving eating disorder treatment because of its calming properties. Additionally for those in residential treatment, I noticed that patients enjoy the comfort of blankets or other sensory soothing items during group sessions or meetings. For some, it may be an interesting skill to learn to knit while in treatment. However if this is too overwhelming, alternatively learning to knit through the use of a loom can be easier and just as beneficial. The beauty of this project is the comfort it can provide not only while making it but once its completed too.

Description: Two Opposing Feelings

Supplies: Drawing Paper (to be folded in half), Pencil, Eraser, Chalk or Oil Pastels, Markers, and Colored Pencils

Directions: Dialectical Behavior Therapy is a useful and frequently used therapeutic model in the treatment of eating disorders. Dialectics refer to two opposing feelings that can both be true and occur at the same time (Linehan, 2014). In this directive, patients are asked to think of a current dialectic that they may be struggling with or working on. Specifically relating to eating disorder recovery, patients may choose something like "being afraid of change and wanting to recover." Patients may have various nuances related to recovery to explore or even a relationship dynamic affected by the disease.

Reference List

Hinz, L. (2006). *Drawing from within: Using art to treat eating disorders*. London: Jessica Kingsley Publishers.

Linehan, M. (2014). *DBT skills training manual*. New York, NY: The Guilford Press.

Chapter 9

Eco-Art

Eco-art therapy, or the incorporation of nature into art therapy work, is of particular interest to me because of my personal love of nature and also because it was the focus of my graduate thesis. Nature can be integrated through the use of materials from nature, making art in nature, or with nature as the subject matter. My graduate thesis explored the use of natural materials in a locked psychiatric unit where patients had limited access to the outdoors. I facilitated art therapy sessions using natural materials and traditional art materials and explored the results. There is a multitude of research showing us that time spent in or near nature has many healing properties. Possibly the most noteworthy study by Dr. Roger Ulrich (1984) found that patients in the hospital who had a window-facing nature recovered faster and needed less pain medication than those facing a brick wall. When I worked for several years in an in-patient psychiatric hospital in Brattleboro, Vermont, I continuously advocated for time outside for patients and integrated eco-art therapy as much as possible into my work there. It is also important to note that for some people, especially those from urban areas, they may not find nature healing but rather uncomfortable. However, I believe, at a primitive level, that nature is something that all our souls desire, and eco-art therapy can be in a less intimidating way to incorporate nature into a person's wellness.

Further Reading: For more in-depth work in the field of eco-art therapy, I suggest the book *Eco-Art Therapy in Practice* by Amanda Alders Pike (2021).

Description: Collaborative Sculpture

Supplies: Space in Nature

Directions: For this group project, I find it useful to show clients artwork by Andy Goldsworthy and other nature-based artists for inspiration. Ask the group to work collaboratively and create a sculptural piece using only materials from nature around them. This can be challenging for groups that are not cohesive or if patients or residents are not getting along, as with any group rapport directives. Lastly, I ask the group to title the piece before we process together what it was like for them.

DOI: 10.4324/9781003413363-9

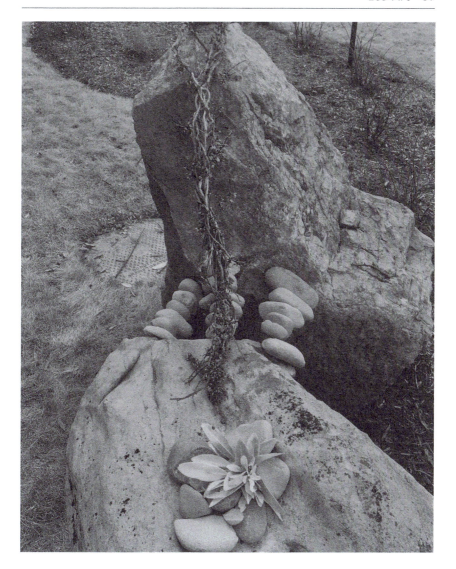

Figure 9.1 Collaborative Eco-Art Sculpture.

Source: Photograph by the author.

Description: Personal Connection to Nature

Supplies: Air Dry Clay or Canvas Boards, Acrylic Paint, Acrylic Paint Brushes, Paint Palette, Water Cup, and Paper Towel

Directions: Ask clients to think of an animal, plant, or perhaps place in nature that they feel deeply connected to. Clients can use any two or three dimensional medium to create this. I have found it particularly interesting in a group format to refine it to animals and have group members sculpt the animal using clay. At the conclusion, when clients are processing their artwork, they can discuss what characteristics about this animal they connect with and why it is significant to them.

Video: This directive can also be explained through a video format. Please see https://www.youtube.com/watch?v=cWz1G_zjY8M&t=180s for a video explanation on the William & Mary Health and Wellness YouTube.

Description: Rock Art

Supplies: An Assortment of Rocks, Acrylic Paint, Paint Palette, Paint Brushes, Acrylic Paint Pens, Water Cup, and Paper Towel

Directions: In this directive I like to incorporate mindfulness by asking clients to really slow down and notice the shape and details of the rock they selected before painting it. After doing so, clients are asked to create something based on the shape of the rock. Often I will also have clients use a paint pen to perhaps write a significant word on the back that might bring them a sense of calm or whatever the particular goal of the group or session is.

Important Note: From past experience, this exercise can take time or more than one session because of the three dimensional nature of rocks. Sometimes clients can struggle to paint both sides or get a base coat within a short time period due to paint drying time.

Description: Rock Wrapping

Supplies: Smaller Rocks of Various Sizes, Yarn, Jute, Leather or Other Fibers for Wrapping the Rocks, and Assorted Additional Natural Materials

Directions: This directive really accentuates the beauty of all things natural and again can be incorporated into mindfulness practices. Have clients begin by selecting materials to work with. Each person will need: a rock, a type of fiber for wrapping, and maybe an additional natural element to enhance. Clients then begin by wrapping the rock with the fiber or string short ways. Sometimes I even use a small amount of tape to hold down the first piece on what will be the backside of the rock. Next this can be looped at the center on the front or wrapped around the other natural element such as a feather or piece of lavender. Continue on with this process so that it continues down the entire length of the front side of the rock. Be sure to secure the ends with small knots or by tucking on the backside of the rock.

Video: This directive in particular can best be explained through a video format. Please see https://www.youtube.com/watch?v=P2n3oSjvhm0 for a video explanation on the William & Mary Health and Wellness YouTube.

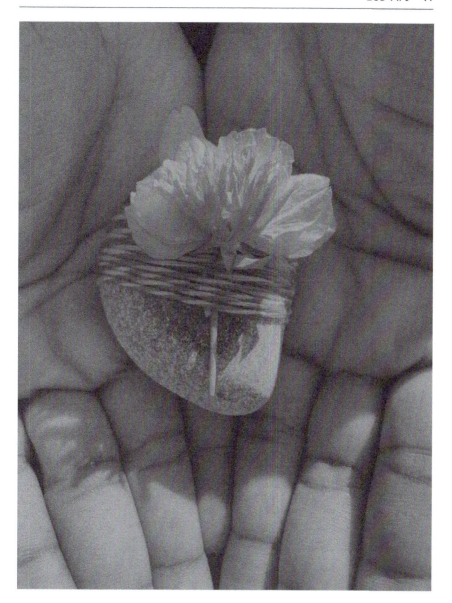

Figure 9.2 Rock Wrapping.

Source: Photograph by the author.

Contraindicated: This can exercise is advanced and can be challenging for those who get easily frustrated or may struggle with fine motor skills.

Reference List

Pike, A. A. (2021). *Eco-art therapy in practice*. New York, NY: Routledge.

Ulrich, R. S. (1984). View through a window may influence recovery from surgery. *Science. 224*(4647), 420–421. doi: 10.1126/science.6143402.

Chapter 10

Emotion Recognition

Paul Cezanne once said, "A work of art which did not begin in emotion is not art." The painter Louis Bourgeois was quoted as saying, "An artist can show things that other people are terrified of expressing." The prolific Pablo Picasso famously said, "Art washes away from the soul the dust of everyday life." There are plentiful amounts of words, writings, and famous quotes about the connection between emotions and art making that span time. It is often hard to tell which came first – the emotion or the art? Many times we have emotions that are difficult to express, but once we start making art, it becomes clearer. On the other hand, if we simply begin making art, emotions arise. I recall one particular peer supervision session where we decided to just start making art without even starting with any type of conversation. A professional trigger for me was recalled, and all the deeply connected emotions became clearer. This in turn helped me realize what in the professional situation was troubling me and I could then let it go. This may be common occurrence for those of us who are naturally inclined to the creative arts or for those of us who are good at expressing ourselves. However, recognizing and expressing emotions does not come easy for all of us. This is another area where I see art therapy especially helpful. It can make it easier for those who struggle to express their emotions because of its less direct nature. Recognizing and identifying emotions is an important skill for children and people of any age in order to live a full and functional life. Beginning by identifying different emotions and how they feel inside our bodies is the first step. Once we are able to recognize emotions, it is then another challenge to learn how to deal with them and/or express them in a healthy way. One way of tapping into our feelings, whether they are big or more subtle, is through art making. Additionally, feeling all of the various emotions good and bad is what makes up life. Understanding emotions is a therapeutic topic that is important to many different client needs, ages, and diagnoses. Below are some art therapy interventions that I have used that are helpful in working with the expression of various emotions.

DOI: 10.4324/9781003413363-10

Description: Emotions Character Sculpture

Supplies: White or Colored Air Dry Clay (Model Magic® is my preference for this project), Washable Markers, and Black Permanent Marker

Directions: I was inspired by the animated movie "*Inside Out*" for this art therapy directive. Based on which emotion your client may be working on, ask them to create a character who embodies this emotion. Have clients begin by wedging the clay in their hands or on the table in front of them to warm it up. Next have clients roll out the clay and they can give it color by drawing onto the clay with washable markers. Then they will mash it up and blend it over and over until the desired color is. Have clients think about the color of the character, for example red for anger or green for jealousy. They can think about other characteristics of this emotion character that they could portray. They could also give the character a name. Depending on the particular focus of the work for the client, they could imagine what it might be like to be this character or even do some role play with it.

Description: Emotion Painting

Supplies: Watercolor, Tempera, or Acrylic Paint, Paint Palette, Paint Brushes, Canvas or Watercolor Paper, Water Cup, and Paper Towel

Directions: For those who struggle to understand different emotions and expressing them, this is a good exercise. Have clients pick or perhaps the therapist suggests a particular emotion for the client to focus on. Maybe this is one they are currently working on or may push away. I also usually have on hand a long list of numerous different emotions for clients to utilize more nuanced feelings words. Ask the client to paint what this emotion might look like. I encourage clients to mostly use colors, lines, and shapes to represent this emotion, rather than realistic symbols. Sometimes clients will intermix a couple different emotions they may be feeling at the same time.

Variation: This is also a particularly effective group directive and group members can try to figure out what emotion each person was trying to convey as clients process their art work.

Description: Emotions Wheel

Supplies: Mixed Media Paper, Acrylic Paints, Paint Palette, Paint Brushes, Water Cup, and Paper Towels

Directions: Psychologist Robert Plutchik created the Wheel of Emotions to organize and explain how the numerous emotions humans can experience are all related. It is a helpful way to decipher subtle variations in emotions

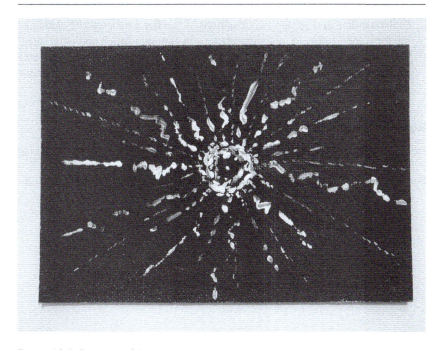

Figure 10.1 Painting of Anxiety.
Source: Photograph by Lindsay Heck and artwork by the author.

especially for those who tend to express big emotions. I begin this art therapy directive by giving some background and psycho education about the Emotions Wheel. Then using mixed media paper and acrylic paints, ask clients to create their own emotions wheel but with the same basic central emotions: joy, trust, fear, surprise, sadness, disgust anger, and anticipation (2002). Clients can explore paint colors and how they may represent these emotions. They can also use their own words to create the various intensities on the spectrum of each of these primary emotions. This emotions wheel can then be a tool that is kept to work with in future sessions or as a reference point for the client at home.

Description: Facial Expressions

Supplies: One-Half of a Face Portrait Photocopied, Pencil, Eraser, Blending Stick, and Charcoal Sticks

Directions: A traditional teaching technique for drawing is to complete the other half of a photocopy of a face. I thought of this technique as a way to recognize subtleties of a person's facial expressions and emotions.

Understanding and recognizing emotions in another person can be challenging for some leading to misinterpretations in communication and other interpersonal challenges. When working in great detail to replicate the other half of a face, it can really teach us to pick up on small nuances like the corners of the mouth turning up or down and slight changes in the eyes.

Reference List

Doctor, P., & Del Carmen, R. (2015). *Inside out*. Emeryville, CA: Pixar Animation Studios.

Plutchik, R. (2002). *Emotions and life: Perspectives from psychology, biology, and evolution*. Washington DC: American Psychological Association.

Chapter 11

Families

Family art therapy is a standard practice in residential treatment centers or is often requested in private practice. It is such a complex subfield of art therapy and traditional psychotherapy that many practitioners usually specialize in or get additional training in this field. Art therapy can be particularly useful in family work because it can add a point of focus for challenging family dynamics. Many times family members can be resistant, tense, or generally not familiar with therapy and the art can ease this. My first art therapy internship was at a halfway house for women and children working through family reunification after custody being taken away due to addiction. We utilized family art therapy as a way to work on facilitating the parent and child connection after being separated from one another for over a year. Not only did the art making provide a point of focus for the session in a highly emotional and tense circumstance, but it was also a parenting skill. Our family art therapy sessions helped the mother to learn skills for engaging with her child in a different way than she had previously. After more than a year apart, the child had developed and changed quite a bit and making art together was a way for the two of them to bond and connect with one another. This is just one case example that describes some aspects of the effectiveness of family art therapy. Below are a few brief family oriented art therapy exercises, but as I stated earlier, I wholly recommend specialized training or continuing education in this field.

Further Reading: Helen Landgarten (1987) was a pioneer in the field of art therapy specializing in family work. Her book, *Family Art Psychotherapy: A Clinical Guide And Casebook*, is an essential read for all art therapists.

Description: Collaborative Painting

Supplies: 18 × 24 or Greater Sized Canvas, Acrylic Paints, Paint Palette, Paint Brushes, Water Cup, and Paper Towels

Directions: A stimulating directive to better understand family dynamics is a collaborative group painting with all the family members. In this directive,

DOI: 10.4324/9781003413363-11

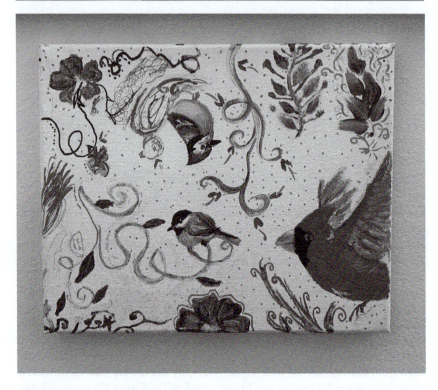

Figure 11.1 Collaborative Painting.
Source: Photograph by the author.

the theme of the painting can be selected by the family or the therapist. Family members are asked to work together on one canvas using acrylic paint. It is interesting to note whether each person uses a certain side or if they all intermingle their boundaries. I often challenge family members to interact in some way with each other on the canvas. Lastly ask the family to come up with a title when they feel it is complete.

Description: Family Portrait

Supplies: Drawing Paper, Crayons, Colored Pencils, Markers, Oil or Chalk Pastels

Directions: Seemingly very simple, family portraits can lead to meaningful discussions in a family session. Family members can each draw their own family portrait or they can create one collectively. Ask clients to also put the family in a memorable place or at home.

Note: Although similar, this is directive is not the Kinetic Family Art Therapy Drawing Technique, which requires a different style of training.

Description: Favorite Memory

Supplies: Drawing Paper for Each Family Member, Crayons, Colored Pencils, Markers, Oil or Chalk Pastels

Directions: In an effort to focus on the positive connections in a family session, I have used this directive. Ask each family member to think independently about a positive memory they have as a family and draw these on their own separate sheets of paper. Processing these images is where the important work takes place and can be a reminder to family members of positive experiences they have had and could potentially build upon for their future.

Description: Genogram

Supplies: Drawing Paper, Pencil, Eraser, Colored Pencil, Fine Point Markers, and Air Dry Clay (Model Magic® is my preference for this project)

Directions: This can be done together collaboratively as a group or separately depending on the specific goal of the family session. Genograms are a pictorial representation of a family's lineage. Often this could include relationship strains, divorces, medical and psychological diagnoses as well as details about relatives ages or birth and death dates. These can be made as creatively as the family is interested in doing. They are particularly helpful in understanding family history, dynamics, and common patterns.

Variation 1: A variation of the traditional family genogram could be to create a symbol to represent each family member that is particular to their personality or interests or more specifically each relative could be a different animal.

Variation 2: Additionally, this could be made out of play dough or clay to add a tactile element for younger children.

Reference List

Landgarten, H. (1987). *Family art psychotherapy: A clinical guide and casebook.* New York, NY: Routledge.

Chapter 12

Grief

I struggled to start to write this chapter, probably because it reminds me of the grief I worked through losing my parents, but also because of the "stuckness" that loss can feel like. Similar to trauma, grief work seems to be felt in the body, often a loss for words that only the creative arts can touch. Grief is most often thought of literally, relating to the death of a loved one. However, it can also take shape more broadly, such as the loss of the idea of something in particular, moving, divorce, layoffs, or an element of a person's identity that may have shifted. Healing from grief takes time, and so does art making. The below directives and mediums I have selected offer a sense of honoring the past. Also important, the artwork created in these directives can provide a sort of transitional object to the late person. After a certain amount of time, I have found that these objects or memories actually bring a sense of warmth and connection rather than sorrow. I would like to dedicate this chapter to my late parents.

Description: Embroidery Memory

Supplies: Embroidery Ring, Fabric, Embroidery Floss, Needles, and Scissors

Directions: Just the idea of embroidery seemingly conjures up feelings of warm memories. In this directive, clients can select a quote or symbol that reminds them of their loved one that has passed. The art piece can then become a wall hanging or pillow as a comforting symbol in the loving memory of the client's beloved person.

Description: Ornament

Supplies: Clear Plastic Ball Ornaments, Memorabilia of the Loved One, and Ribbon

Directions: For this art therapy directive, the client will need a clear plastic ball ornament. These can be purchased online or at any craft supply store. The holidays are a particularly difficult time of year after we have lost a

DOI: 10.4324/9781003413363-12

loved one. In this exercise, clients can store small keepsakes from the person they are grieving and put them inside the clear plastic ornament. Items can include: old letters or recipes, photos, charms, or other small but important mementos. Lastly tie a decorative ribbon for the ornament to be hung from.

Description: Letting Go Leaves

Supplies: Mixed Media Paper, Scissors, Colored Pencils, Markers, Fine Point Permanent Pens, Pastels, Watercolor Pencil, Watercolor Brushes, Water Cup, and Paper Towel

Directions: The cyclical rhythm of the seasons can provide a healing parallel to life, death, and grief. This directive can be a traditional grief exercise or rather about loss and or letting go in a more broad sense. Clients begin by selecting a leaf or petal form to either trace from (a premade template) or create their own. Clients can then use watercolor, colored pencils, or pastel to add color to the one side of the leaf. On the back or integrated into the piece, ask clients to write something they would like to "let go of."

Description: Origami Crane

Supplies: Origami Paper and Pencil

Directions: Origami the Japanese art form of folding paper and has a particularly mindful quality to it that many find soothing. The origami crane above all is known as a symbol of healing. I begin by asking clients to write a

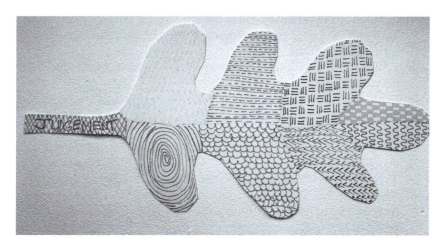

Figure 12.1 Letting Go Leaf (with Template).
Source: Photograph and artwork by the author.

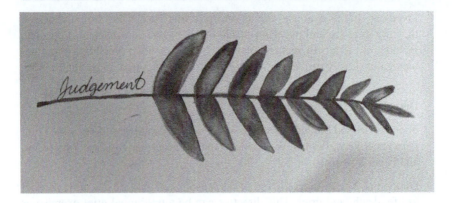

Figure 12.2 Letting Go Leaf.

Source: Photograph and artwork by the author.

hope or a wish on the plain side of the origami paper. Then we usually work together or in a group on the step-by-step folds. Lastly during the processing portion of the group, clients would share their wish or hope and how it may relate to their grief work.

Steps:

- Begin with the decorative side of the paper face down on the table and the white side face up.
- Place the paper so that it is in a diamond shape in front of you.
- I like to use cardinal directions when explaining origami steps.
- Next fold the top point (North) to the bottom point (South).
- Then fold the East side to meet the West side and you should now have a triangle on a right angle.
- Take the Southern corner and separate the two layers of sheets and flatten it into a square.
- Flip it over and do the same thing on that side creating a smaller diamond shape.
- Next is the trickiest part where people can easily become frustrated. Take the top layer and lift it backwards flattening it into an elongated diamond shape.
- Then flip it over and create the same elongated diamond shape on this side.
- Now take the east side of the elongated diamond and folded toward the center line.
- Again do the same thing on the West side of the elongated diamond.
- Lastly we will create the wings by folding the top triangles down.
- Finally create the head and tail from the two smaller last pieces.

Video: For a step-by-step video I created on the William & Mary Health and Wellness YouTube channel please see https://www.youtube.com/watch?v= M-Qli9BtCXc&t=24s.

Variation: During the pandemic when I was mainly facilitating art therapy over zoom and client's at home supplies were limited, I would have clients make their own origami paper. I have now incorporated this into this directive when appropriate. Clients can cut paper into a square shape and draw some type of repetitive decorative design on one side of the paper. It is still important to keep one side plain to help with folding instructions.

Contraindicated: Origami is not for everyone because of its step-by-step exacting nature and can easily frustrate younger clients or those with motor issues. This can lead to the client thinking more about their seeming lack of skill rather than the actual grief work.

Chapter 13

Group Rapport

When I switched careers from in-patient hospitals and residential work to providing art therapy at a university wellness center, there was a big shift in focus from acute care to prevention work. Group rapport is important in both areas of art therapy work, no matter the level of acuity. However, an important distinction is whether or not clients will be seeing each other in a longer term living situation or on the other end of the spectrum, where colleagues might hardly know each other. Graduate-level art therapists will begin their experience through internships and usually early career work for art therapists is in some type of group setting and so therefore understanding group dynamics is essential. Below are a few group rapport-building art therapy directives that can be used with various acuity levels and adapted as needed by the art therapist.

Description: Group Art

Supplies: Large White Paper Roll or Large Canvas, Pencil, Eraser, Pastels, Markers, Acrylic Paint, Acrylic Paint Brushes, Paint Palette, Water Cup, and Paper Towels

Directions: For this art therapy directive, focused on group dynamics, participants need to be stable enough or have enough rapport to tolerate others working closely or potentially on top of their own art work. I generally use this directive as a concluding session for a group. In the past, I have rolled out a large sheet of paper covering the table or cut it into a circle to create a group mandala. In smaller groups (and when budget allows) I have used a large canvas and had groups paint collaboratively on it. This collaborative art can have a certain theme related to the focus of the group or generally about termination. I usually "challenge" the group and ask them to interact in some way with the other group members. An example could be, if someone has drawn a flower another member could add a bee landing on it. However it could equally be used as an introductory get-to-know-you session.

DOI: 10.4324/9781003413363-13

Note: Be mindful that some group projects cannot be taken home by participants. In some cases, participants can cut a portion of the piece to take home
or take a photo of the piece.

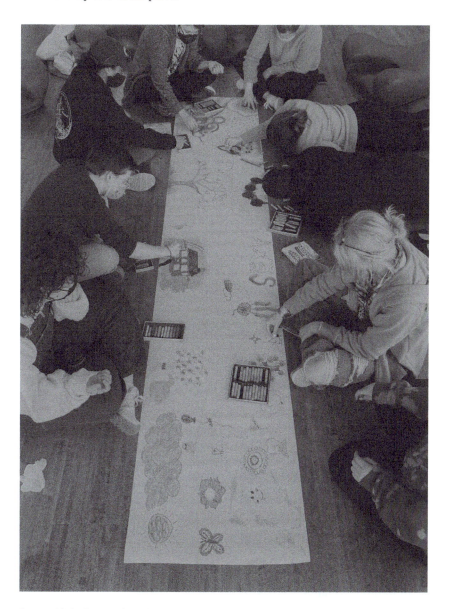

Figure 13.1 Group Art Making.

Source: Photograph by the author.

Description: Mini-Canvas Collab

Supplies: 3 × 3 Mini Canvases, Acrylic Paints, Paint Palette, Paint Brushes, Water Cup, and Paper Towels

Directions: When working on group rapport building, collaborative art making is great way to connect group members by having them work together. Begin by having the group decide on a complete image or theme for the group collaborative painting. This could be a symbol relating to the purpose of the particular group. Next each participant uses their own mini-square canvas to piece together one larger image. This will take team work to line up the parts just right so that it looks like one complete image all together.

Description: Round Robin

Supplies: Drawing Paper, Pencil, Eraser, Markers, or Colored Pencils

Directions: I learned this staple art therapy directive in my graduate program at Pratt Institute. Each participant begins with a paper and something to draw with. As with all directives, the art therapist can lead as much as is necessary for that particular session. I usually start with the prompt, "draw a being of some sort." Examples could include an alien, horse, teacher, etc. Participants then pass their paper to the person next to them and that person needs to then add something and so on for as many rounds are fitting for that session. The art therapist can be as involved with the various prompts for each round as is appropriate. It is exciting at the end during processing for participants to all show their drawings. They all will have the same elements, but the completed drawings will likely look somewhat different. Be sure to return the starting image to the first person who initiated it.

Contraindicated: As with the previous group directive, participants need to be stable enough to accept other people drawing on their art work. Also for residential settings where complicated interpersonal dynamics form, an exercise like this may not be clinically appropriate.

Variations: For an individual session rather than with groups, this could also be done simply between the therapist and the client one on one in a back and forth manner. I have also found that this directive translates really well over virtual sessions which you will see below in Chapter 30: Virtual Art Therapy.

Description: Shapes Match Up

Supplies: 11 × 18 Drawing Paper, Scissors, Masking Tape, Pencil, Eraser, Markers, or Colored Pencils

Directions: I learned this art therapy directive in my graduate art education program at Lesley University. Prior to the session, the art therapist needs to cut the papers in half short ways but in varying ways such as: zigzag, wavy, keyhole, etc. Put an "x" on the backside of the matching pieces to make sure they will line up for the ending of this directive. Make sure there are enough halves for each group member and if it is an odd number of participants, then the art therapist will need to create one as well. Randomly place one at people's spots or hand out the varying shapes to all the group members as they arrive. Encourage participants to turn the paper in several directions until they see something they could draw that fills the shape of the paper. (Important note: the paper can be turned in any direction but only drawn on the blank side, not the side with the "x".) After group members have filled their page, ask them to find their matching half. In partners, they can then attach their two pieces together on the back with the masking tape, discuss it, and title it if desired.

Chapter 14

LGBTQIA+

As a cisgender straight woman, I have a lot to learn about the LGBTQIA+ community and the oppression and mental health struggles they face. Previously, I worked at a psychiatric hospital in Brattleboro, Vermont, where there is a unit specific to the mental health issues that may arise as a queer individual. One piece of data that I recall standing out to me is that LGBTQIA+ adults and youth are more than twice as likely to experience mental health struggles, yet more than 60% were not able to receive adequate treatment (Nami, 2023; The Trevor Project, 2022). As with other sub-specialties, I would encourage additional training in this field, as I have found that helpful for myself. I am certainly not an expert, but all therapists should be able to work with LGBTQIA+ clients in today's world to create a safe, affirming space and use current, inclusive language. I have been an ally through holding private sessions for various LGBTQIA+ student organizations at the university where I work, and I am grateful to have been given this opportunity and will continue to.

Further Reading: While research and writing on art therapy with the LGBTQIA+ community is limited, I recommend the book *Creative Arts Therapies and the LGBTQ Community: Theory and Practice* by MacWilliam, Harris, Trottier, and Long.

Description: Altered Bookmaking

Supplies: Used Books, Collage Magazines and Scrap Paper, Scissors, Glue Sticks, Pencil, Eraser, Colored Pencils, Fine Point Permanent Markers, and Pens

Directions: Altered books, the technique of making art onto a book, is adaptable to any art therapy directive but I have found it particularly meaningful when working with LGBTQIA+ groups or individuals. The actual book that the client works on may be specific to the theme of the client's work or not. There is something that feels rebellious or perhaps even corrective about re-writing a story or altering it. Clients can use various art mediums and techniques to create art onto the book and there are endless amounts of

DOI: 10.4324/9781003413363-14

information about this online. Often altered book projects are on-going and something that clients can continue with after the sessions have ended even.

Description: Pride Buttons

Supplies: Button Making Supplies, Drawing Paper, Scissors, Pencil, Eraser, Fine Point Permanent Markers, and Colored Pencils

Directions: I have used this directive for sessions focused on advocacy. Button making supplies can be purchased at art supply stores and online, coming with a front and back that can be snapped together usually coming in bulk with varying sizes. Clients begin by tracing the smaller half of the two button parts, this is important or it will be too large and warp the paper once put

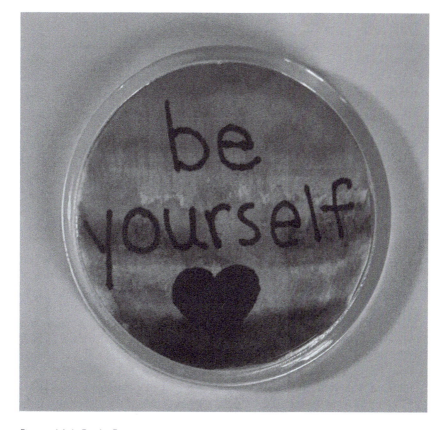

Figure 14.1 Pride Button.
Source: Photograph by the author.

together. Using any two dimensional materials, clients can create any sort of image or messaging they feel is important. These can be for the client themselves or maybe even for family members or other allies to wear or display.

Description: Rainbow Yarn Wrapping

Supplies: Yarn in Red, Orange, Yellow, Green, Blue, Violet, and Scissors

Directions: "In 1978, Gilbert Baker of San Francisco designed and made a flag with six stripes representing the six colors of the rainbow as a symbol of gay and lesbian community pride" (Alyson Almanac, 1989). This is now a celebrated symbol for the diverse people that make up the LGBTQIA+ community. Whether as a member of this community or as an ally, clients may begin the process of wanting to show a sense of pride. There are a number of rainbow items that one can purchase, but it is even more powerful when we make them ourselves or in a group with the same mission. Yarn wrapping is a fiber arts technique that is a simple but mindful process. Everyday items such as phone or computer chargers, keychains, or water bottles can be wrapped in rainbow yarn as a symbol seen every day for LGBTQIA+ pride. These could also be gifts for family members and allies leading to important discussions.

Variation: For a group with an LGBTQIA+ mission 'yarn bombing' could be a powerful exercise to work collaboratively on. Considered to be one of the developers of this technique, Magda Sayeg uses yarn bombing or yarn wrapping on large scale everyday items in our environment. Sayeg (2023) explains, "I love displacing hand made, mostly woven, material in environments where it seemingly doesn't belong... only to discover that they can coexist quite harmoniously... The exploration of environmental change drives me: provoking the world to be a more challenging, unconventional, and interesting place." When we did a yarn bombing installation at the university where I work, we needed to obtain clearance and permission. While this technique is traditionally done more in a surprise graffiti-style, that is of course not appropriate for a therapeutic group and therefore proper permissions should be attained before beginning. Next decide on a meaningful place for the yarn bombing. This group exercise will likely last more than the usual one hour session timeframe depending on the scale of the project which is why it is also important to think about when figuring out a location. The technique of yarn wrapping is just as it sounds, where you wrap the item with yarn row by row close enough together that the original color cannot be seen below until it is completely covered. When changing colors to create a rainbow affect, simply attach the transitioning colors together with a secure knot.

Description: Song Lyric or Quote

Supplies: Small Canvases, Pencil, Eraser, Fine Point Permanent Marker, Acrylic Paint, Paint Palette, Paint Brushes, Water Cup, and Paper Towel

Directions: As with many of these art therapy directives, this one can also be applied to various types of sessions. Ask the client or group members to think of an impactful song lyric or quote that relates to the focus of their work. Clients may want to do this before the session as "homework" in preparation for this directive. Previously my clients have enjoyed working on small 8 × 5 or rectangular canvases to display these pieces in their spaces at home. Clients can paint abstractly the background and use fine point marker to write the quote or any portion of it on top. These pieces can be displayed or used as an affirmation to the client.

Reference List

Almanac, A. (1989). *Alyson almanac: A treasury of information for the gay and lesbian community*. New York, NY: Alyson Books.

MacWilliam, B., Harris, B. T., Trottier, D. G., & Long, K. (2022) *Creative arts therapies and the LGBTQ community: Theory and practice*. London: Jessica Kingsley Publishers.

NAMI. (2023). *LGTBQI*. Retrieved from https://www.nami.org/Your-Journey/Identity-and-Cultural-Dimensions/LGBTQI.

Sayeg, M. (2023). *Magda Sayeg*. Retrieved from http://www.magdasayeg.com.

The Trevor Project. (2022). *National Survey on LGTBQ Youth Mental Health*. Retrieved from https://www.thetrevorproject.org/survey-2022/#intro.

Chapter 15

Life Transitions

At some point in every person's life span, they will go through a challenging transition. Examples of this could include: entering college, relationship break-ups, moving, changing careers, marriages, divorces, aging, retirement, and other milestones. As with other art therapy directives in this book, many in this section can be altered or used in varying ways to suit your particular client circumstance. I recall one particular case example where the art therapy truly expressed the client's transitional process. The client was struggling particularly with coming of age, independence, and confidence around her self-actualization process. When we first began working together, her artwork, no matter which medium she would choose, was always very pale in color. If it was watercolor, the paints would be very watered down. If it was pencil, she would press very lightly. If it was acrylic paint, she would mix a lot of white into all the pigments. As we continued to work together and she gained more and more self-assurance, I noticed her artwork became more and more vibrant. This was a visual recording of her own growth through the art making. Not only was it a beautiful process to watch as an art therapist, but also something significant for her to reflect back on afterward. Life transitions like this one I described can occur at any stage of the life span, so it is useful for the practicing art therapist to have experience and specific projects dedicated to this area. Another significant life transition is the process of leaving to attend college. I have utilized most of these art therapy directives below, particularly with the college students I work with at the university where I work, as they blossom into their independent adulthood, but many can be adapted to various life stages.

Description: Acceptance Art

Supplies: Air Dry Clay, Clay Tools, and Water Cup

Directions: Marsha Linehan (2014) says, "Acceptance is the only way out of hell." This is the basis for her revolutionary theory called Radical Acceptance. When unlucky or bad things happen to people, we inevitably begin with

DOI: 10.4324/9781003413363-15

questioning, 'why me?!' Radical Acceptance is the idea that by whole-heartedly accepting whatever horrible has happened to us, we will then begin to heal and reduce mal-adaptive behaviors. For this directive, ask clients to create an image or clay sculpture of what it feels like to fight or deny whatever it is that has happened to them. Then create a second piece of what it may look like to accept it. The client may not even be able to conjure an image yet for this, but can eventually work towards it. Clay can be an interesting medium for this exercise because it can provide a sense of response to the client or a parallel process of pushing back.

Description: Draw Yourself on a Path

Supplies: Drawing Paper, Pencil, Eraser, Colored Pencil, Markers, or Pastels

Directions: This classic art therapy directive may get clients to think more closely about what they have been through and where they are going. Ask clients to think about where they might currently be on any sort of path or route. The actual surroundings for this drawing are up to them. I usually encourage clients to think about things like whether the environment is safe or rugged. Maybe they are in the middle of a challenging course or they have just arrived at the top of an uphill battle. In the past, clients have added other surrounding elements like certain animals, weather, or environmental factors. Lastly, the client can then place themselves along this path somewhere in a realistic or symbolic way.

Description: Guided Imagery

Supplies: Air Dry Clay or Drawing Paper, Pencil, Eraser, Markers, or Pastels

Directions: Guided imagery can be a useful tool for those needing to listen to their intuition. Often when people are going through a life transition, important decisions may be part of the process. Just as valuable as a "pros and cons" list, however guided imagery can provide answers through a person's inner wisdom. There are many resources for guided imagery scripts, but for this purpose I usually select one that involves some kind of journey and ending with a final answer or image that appears for the client. I then ask clients to create art to represent what they saw at the conclusion of the guided meditation. Below is a guided meditation I have used for this exercise written by Susi McWilliam (2022) from her book *35 Guided Meditation Scripts: Scripts for Meditation Teachers, Yoga Teachers, Therapists, Coaches, Counsellors and Healers* which I recommend.

Breathing deeply, I want you to now visualize yourself in the most beautiful garden. You look around the garden and see all the signs of spring around you see daffodils growing a black bird pecking for worms and you can hear the low buzz about bumblebee in the distance. You notice butterflies dancing from flower to flower then you feel the gentle warmth of the sun on your face this is your own special garden, a place where you can plant your hopes and dreams a place where you can feel calm and safe.

You notice a greenhouse at the end of the garden and you begin to walk towards it. You can feel the warmth as you open the greenhouse door and inside you notice a packet of seeds. You pick up this packet of seeds and head back out to your beautiful garden. In your garden there's a patch of nourishing deep earthy compost. You use a trowel and make some small holes in that compost. The compost and patch of earth is where you can plant your dreams.

I'd like you to now take one seed from your packet and think of something you wish to grow what do you wish to bring into your life? And you breathe in feeling the sun on your face and place your hands in the earthy soil and plant that hope and dream into your patch. You lovingly cover it with some compost and move forward to the next hole that you've made you feel a sense of satisfaction and joy in your heart, and you're excited about new beginnings and opportunities you take the next seed from the packet and place it gently in the hole, and with it, place your hopes, your dreams. You continue to do this with other seeds for things you wish to retain in your life the things you wish to nourish, relationships, hobbies. Whatever you want to bring into your life and you want to nourish and grow, plant the seeds of those in your patch when you're finished, you gently pat the ground. You notice a watering can beside the patch and use it to sprinkle water you feel fulfilled, calm, peaceful. You pause to take one last look around your garden.

You notice the buds within the trees, the leaves beginning to appear on bushes and pansies beginning to grow along the path. You're filled with a sense of hope. Because just as nature changes and grows from season to season, so do you. With every day with every moment, in fact with every breath you take, there is an opportunity. The opportunity to start afresh. The opportunity for new beginnings. An opportunity to nourish and give gratitude for all the magnificent things you always have you already have in your life.

Contraindicated: Guided imagery is not recommended for clients or patients who are not cognitively present for reasons such as psychosis or dementia.

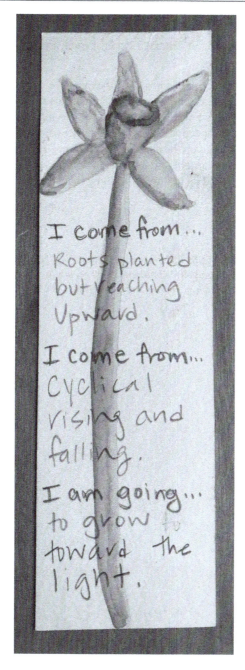

Figure 15.1 *"I Come From"* Art Journaling Example.

Source: Photograph and artwork by the author.

Description: I Come From

Supplies: Art Journals or Drawing Paper, Pencil, Eraser, Pens, and Colored Pencils

Directions: This directive can be used for expressive writing and or visual art. I learned this particular directive in my graduate art therapy program at Pratt Institute. As I recall, we were given options of varying objects and then asked to write from the perspective of this item. In my own work as an art therapist, I have altered it and given the simple prompt of begin writing with the words "I come from." Another alteration that is more focused on visual art than expressive writing could be to draw something that represents where you come from and where you are going.

Reference List

Linehan, M. (2014). *DBT skills training manual*. New York, NY: The Guilford Press.
McWilliam, S. (2022). *35 guided meditation scripts: Scripts for meditation teachers, yoga teachers, therapists, coaches, counsellors and healers*. Aberdeen UK: Self-Published.

Chapter 16

Medical Art Therapy

Another subspecialty in the field of art therapy is the focus on working with those affected by medical illnesses and hospitalizations rather than mental health-related work. I highly recommend advanced training; additionally, there are even art therapy graduate programs that focus specifically on this field. Music therapy is a well-researched and practiced creative arts modality in medically ill and hospice care work. Research by Shella (2018) affirms that art therapy with medically ill hospitalized patients see "significant improvements in pain, mood and anxiety levels after between the start and the end of art therapy sessions." I was afforded the opportunity to volunteer in a medical hospital in Burlington, Vermont, using art with pediatric patients. The joy and distraction it brought to these children was remarkable. Of course, there can be limitations if patients cannot leave their rooms, or perhaps relating to mobility or energy levels, which is why the art therapist needs to be able to adapt quickly. I have found the directives below to be attainable for many to be able to practice in a medical art therapy environment.

Further Reading: For more in-depth reading on the subspecialty of medical art therapy, I recommend the book *Art Therapy and Healthcare* edited by Cathy Malchiodi (2012).

Description: Abstract Self-Portrait

Supplies: Canvas Board, Acrylic Paint, Paint Palette, Paint Brushes, Water Cup, Paper Towel, and Permanent Marker

Directions: When patients are not well they often do not feel like themselves. For this directive, ask patients to create an abstract self-portrait using mixed media. Select a variety of materials for the patient and encourage more abstract representations rather than realistic. Prompt the patient to think about themselves holistically or over a longer period of time, not just as they are right now. The power of positive thinking has long helped many overcome illness and challenging times and if appropriate, maybe the patient could even create a future self-portrait.

DOI: 10.4324/9781003413363-16

Description: Bracelet Weaving

Supplies: Embroidery Floss in Varying Colors, and Scissors

Directions: Weaving with embroidery floss is a well established craft that while most may think is simple, it too has some meditative and calming affects. Similar to knitting, keeping hands busy when nervous is effective and the repetitive nature of the art making process can slow down the body and mind. Once the steps are memorized, a patient can weave in a natural rhythmic way. Another benefit of bracelet weaving is the that takes very minimal materials and can be done almost anywhere which is important in a hospital environment. I have found it helpful to tie the embroidery floss onto something permanent in the environment around the patient. While there are a number of different weaving styles and patterns, I have described below two introductory ones.

Diagonal Pattern:

Begin by taking two arm's lengths of at least three different colors of embroidery floss. Fold the three colors in half so that you now have six strands with a loop at the top. This loop can be attached to anything stable in the patient's environment where they can work from. Begin by deciding on a pattern with the colors. This pattern must stay the same throughout the duration of the weaving. Make the first knot by creating the number four with the first strand over the second strand. Pull this knot to the top and repeat a second time. Take the same strand you begin with and move down to the second piece of embroidery floss. Always making two knots each time and working your way through the entire row of strands of embroidery floss. This strand now becomes the last one in the row. Repeat the same process with the embroidery strand that has moved into the first position in the pattern of colors. It is important to let patients know that it always looks a little uneven and imperfect at the start work, but will begin to form a diagonal repeating pattern as they progress.

Staircase Pattern:

Again, begin by taking two arm's lengths of at least three different colors of embroidery floss. The amount of strands does not really matter for this pattern, but will make it thicker and provide more color options. Fold the strands of embroidery floss in half so that you now have a loop at the top. This loop can be attached to anything stable in the patient's environment where they can work from. Beginning with the strand furthest to the left in the row, make a number four on top of all of the other strands, pull the knot up to the top. Continue to repeat this over and over again and you will notice a staircase pattern begin to form. When the patient would like to change colors, simply switch which strand makes the knot over the rest of the strands.

Description: Dimensions of You

Supplies: Drawing Paper Cut into Circles, Scissors, Ruler (optional), Pencil, Eraser, and Colored Pencils

Directions: First developed by Dr Peggy Swarbrick, the Eight Dimensions of Wellness are a framework for exploring a person's holistic wellness. We utilize this overarching curriculum at the university wellness center where I work. Patients can begin with a piece of pre-cut circular paper or if interested and or beneficial can trace and cut their own circle to start. Have patients divide the circle into eight triangular sections either with a pencil and ruler or by simply folding into eights. Provide psycho education about the different dimensions of wellness (Physical, Mental, Spiritual, Environmental, Social, Financial, Intellectual, and Occupational). It is important to remind clients that this is generally fluctuating, meaning certain areas may be better than others at varying times. Specifically, if the patient's physical wellness is poor right now, what are other dimensions that may be healthier or focused on, for example their spiritual wellness may be stronger. Patients can then create symbols or words in each particular section to represent how they are currently feeling or perhaps goals for that area of their wellness.

Description: Finger Knitting

Supplies: Yarn and Scissors

Directions: As I have previously mentioned, knitting is a helpful medium for anxiety. Being hospitalized and having an illness is most certainly anxiety producing. Finger knitting is an easy coping skill that does not require extensive materials and can be done from a bed or other confined space. Begin by making a slip knot on the thumb of the patient's non-dominant hand. This is just a place holder and can be taken off as progress is made. Next weave the yarn strand through the remaining four fingers in a front, behind, front, behind pattern. After that, wrap the yarn behind and around the entire hand above the finger loops. Then begin to weave, pulling the lower loop over the upper and off each finger, one by one. Continue to repeat by simply wrapping the yarn around the whole hand and then weaving over the fingers. This will form a longer thinner scarf-like shape that can be continued until the desired length is reached. To finish the piece, cut the yarn from the skein and slip it through each finger making a knot on each before taking it off the finger.

Video: This directive in particular can best be explained through a video format. Please see https://www.youtube.com/watch?v=GFmJWUCUhy0&t=25s for a video explanation on the William & Mary Health and Wellness YouTube.

Contraindicated: This can be a challenging fine motor skill which could be a factor for some medically compromised patients.

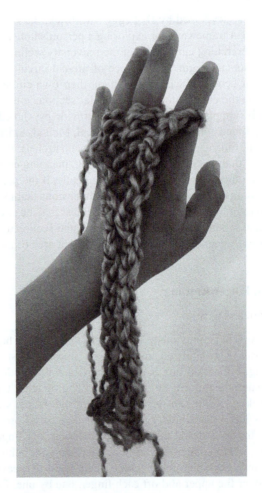

Figure 16.1 Finger Knitting.

Source: Photograph by the author and artwork by Drew Balascio.

Reference List

Malchiodi, C. (Ed.). (2012). *Art therapy and healthcare*. New York, NY: The Guildford Press.

Shella, T. (2018). Art therapy improves mood, and reduces pain and anxiety when offered at bedside during acute hospital treatment. *The Arts in Psychotherapy. 57*, 59–64. doi: 10.1016/j.aip.2017.10.003.

Chapter 17

Mindfulness

Mindfulness is applicable to many different populations, treatment goals, or often used as a daily practice. Mindfulness is staying in the present moment with intention and non-judgmentally (Kabat-Zinn, 1994). I often hear at the end of my art therapy groups that participants find just the simple parts of art making a mindful experience. These are because when we make art we have a tendency to slow down and notice small details in shape and color as we make decisions about what to add or subtract from an art piece. At the McLeod Tyler Wellness Center at the College of William & Mary where I work, I facilitate a Mindful Art Making group. In that group, I often talk with stressed-out college students about when we are rushing around or cramming, it may seem counter-intuitive to make time for something like mindfulness. However, almost all the time, students will say "Wow I was actually better able to focus on my test or writing that paper after practicing mindfulness!" I also usually talk with students about how our minds have a tendency to either jump ahead and worry about the future or perseverate and go over things from the past. These may not necessarily be upsetting thoughts, just benign to-do lists or past conversations. However, the act of staying in the present moment, while challenging, can be really good for our minds and bodies. It can be really powerful for people to know that they have the power to control where their mind goes. We do not have to think about things we do not want to! How great is that to find out! Lastly, in order to notice the progress of how we are feeling in the Mindful Art Group I facilitate, I generally like to have clients write down a few descriptive words about how they are feeling at the start of the session and again at the end because sometimes the differences can be subtle. While in general, art making in many forms can be a mindful experience, below are some specific art therapy directives to help clients stay in the present moment.

Further Reading: For a more in-depth look at the connection between mindfulness and the field of art therapy, I suggest Barbara Jean Davis' *Mindful Art Therapy* (2015).

DOI: 10.4324/9781003413363-17

Description: Drawing Your Breath

Supplies: 11 × 18 or Larger Drawing Paper, Charcoal or Chalk Pastels (or other mediums that are soft or flow easily since eye will be closed or averted)

Directions: Clients are given basic psycho education about mindfulness and breath work to start. Next close your eyes, center yourself, notice your breath. Using chalk pastel and paper align your breath with your marks on the paper. This is best used as a warm up in a session for clients to center themselves and become more present.

Description: Mandala Drawings

Supplies: Drawing Paper Cut into Circles, Pencil, Eraser, Colored Pencils, Pens, Fine Point Markers, Watercolor Pencils, Watercolor Brushes, Water Cup, and Paper Towels

Directions: Clients are given basic psycho education about mindfulness and introduced to what a mandala is. Mandala in Sanskrit translates to circle, and I often discuss the cyclical nature of many things in life and give cultural background as well. I usually have clients note how they are feeling at the start and end of drawing the mandala as it can be centering for people. I also try to have clients focus on creating simple shapes and lines because the typical mandala that people are used to seeing can be overwhelming in their detail for most people. I encourage clients to work from the center outward. Watercolor pencils can be a nice addition to a drawn mandala to fill areas with color.

Note: The Mari Mandala Assessment, a type of clinical evaluation using mandalas, is a much different art therapy techniques than this directive. There are specific trainings and research about this method if art therapists are interested in that instead.

Variation: Group mandala drawings are also interesting especially for building group rapport. Group members each begin their own mandala, then after a set amount of time they pass their mandala to the person next to them to continue working on. I have done this with music in the background as a marker for when to switch mandalas to the person next to them. Group members do need to know ahead of time that their art work will be drawn on by others, which can be challenging for some. However, it is also interesting to see how your mandala has arrived back to you at the end and I find groups members asking each other who added what to their mandalas.

Video: This directive can also be explained through a video format. Please see https://www.youtube.com/watch?v=9usEaR0HpU4&t=385s for a video explanation on the William & Mary Health and Wellness YouTube.

Description: Mindful vs Mind Full

Supplies: Drawing Paper (to be folded in half), Pencil, Eraser, Colored Pencil and Pens

Directions: Clients are given basic psycho education about mindfulness to start. Clients are given paper and fold in half, writing "mindful" on one

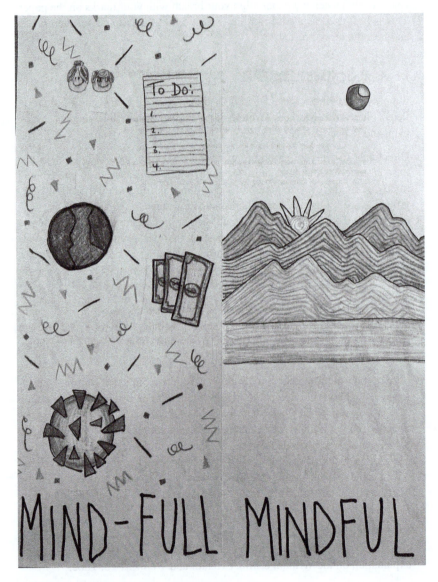

Figure 17.1 Mind-Full versus Mindful Drawing.

Source: Photograph and artwork by the author.

side and "mind full" on the other. Ask clients to think about what fills their minds with clutter, busyness, or perhaps worries. This may or may not be negative thoughts, some may just be neutral or even positive. Then ask clients to compare and think about when they are most mindful or present in their daily lives.

Video: This directive can also be explained through a video format. Please see https://www.youtube.com/watch?v=nbsCw8daF14&t=633s for a video explanation on the William & Mary Health and Wellness YouTube.

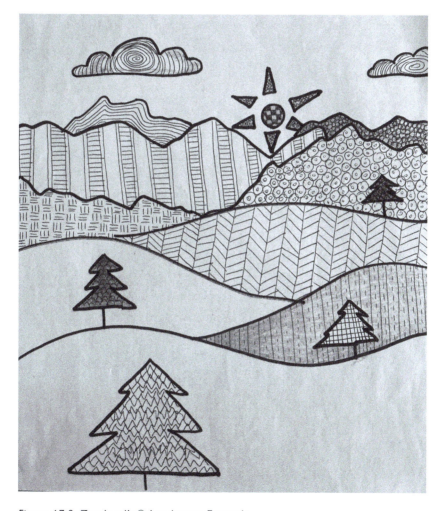

Figure 17.2 Zendoodle® Landscape Example.

Source: Photograph and artwork by the author.

Description: Zendoodles®

Supplies: Mixed Media Paper, Pencil, Eraser, and Colored Pencils (often these are created in black and white, but preference is up to the client)

Directions: Clients are given basic psycho education about mindfulness to start. Zendoodles® are a simple technique of drawing repetitive line patterns within a defined shape or area. These can be abstract, fill an enclosed space, or inside something more realistic as in the image below.

Reference List

Barbara, J. D. (2015). *Mindful art therapy*. London: Jessica Kingsley Publishers.
Kabat-Zinn, J. (1994). *Wherever you go there you are*. New York, NY: Hyperion.

Chapter 18

Multiculturalism

The racial and cultural identity of clients is important to consider for working art therapists, no matter what setting or environment we work in. Unfortunately, for too long, acknowledgment of the lack of considerations for Black, Indigenous, and People of Color in therapy has not been recognized in the field of psychology, and more specifically, art therapy. Research is lacking in the areas of diversity, equity, and social justice in the field of art therapy. Nor is there enough writing or professional training in these fields as well. You will see one excellent book below, but the options are minimal. Without an understanding of where our clients come from and their cultural history, we are missing a large part of the people we are working with. Additionally, our own prejudices and personal experiences may also hinder our perspective and views on our clients as well. Lastly, material choices are also something to consider when selecting art therapy directives as certain mediums may be new or foreign to our clients or rather may make a person more comfortable to utilize in a session. "It is well known that statistics suggest art therapists aren't very ethnically diverse and for many years there has been a desire for cultural approaches that are inclusive of the individuals that engage in art therapy practices" (Jackson, 2020). It is our responsibility as art therapists to educate ourselves and become competent in the most up-to-date and inclusive language and theoretical frameworks when it comes to marginalized and underserved people. Additionally, Tervalon (2015) explains that cultural humility takes it a step further because it is "interconnected with truth, gives power to each voice, is personal, authentic, organic, mutually developed, and skill based… it encompasses partnership, shared decision-making, and is flexible and dynamic" Therefore, art making by the art therapist is also important in sessions. The art therapy directives I have suggested below are focused on cultural diversity and can be completed as a group and include the art therapist as well.

Further Reading: My recommendation for an important book on the topics of privilege, cultural humility, and equity as it relates to the practice of art therapy is called *Cultural Humility in Art Therapy: Applications for Practice, Research, Social Justice, Self-Care, and Pedagogy* by Louvenia Jackson.

DOI: 10.4324/9781003413363-18

Description: Heritage Quilt Squares

Supplies: White Fabric, Variety of Patterned Fabrics, Fabric Markers, Scissors, Needle, and Thread

Directions: This art therapy directive is designed for groups, but there is a variation for individual work below. Each group member can create a square or multiple squares that represent who they are. This could be through fabric colors, prints, or in the pattern style of their heritage. Additionally clients can create their own square by drawing using fabric markers onto plain fabric. Depending on the length and duration of the group, members can collaborate on sewing the squares together. Alternatively the squares can be attached to a line in the style of flags. An important note is that group projects like this are difficult to decide on who gets what portion of it. So it is key to discuss

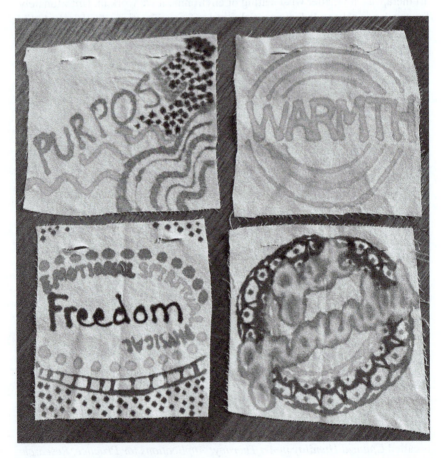

Figure 18.1 Heritage Square Fiber Art.

Source: Photography by the author.

this prior to starting so that clients can be aware they may not get to take what they made home. Also deciding how and where it will be displayed is another essential discussion.

Variation: When working individually on this project, the client could make a few hand drawn squares and intermix in a repeating design with the patterned fabric.

Description: Identity Portrait

Supplies: 8 × 10 or Larger Canvas, Acrylic Paint, Paint Palette, Paint Brushes, Water Cup, and Paper Towels

Directions: Ask the client to think about all the different parts of their identity. This could include- race, gender, societal or family roles, community, family background, heritage, passions, and or spirituality. The idea in this project is not to include an actual visual representation of the client, but the other parts that make up who they are as a person in an abstract art piece. Important note, using acrylic paint on canvas can be challenging for new painters especially when trying to make something realistic or with fine details. If the client chooses to do so, I often encourage participants to sketch it with pencil first and then add the paint in a second step.

Description: Piece of Me

Supplies: Canvas Board or Cardboard, Acrylic Paint, Paint Palette, Water Cup, Paper Towel, Permanent Marker, Scissors, Tissue Paper, Glue Stick, Decoupage Glue and Brush (Mod Podge® is my preference for this project), Important Memorabilia, Photo Copy Machine

Directions: For this directive, the client will highlight an important object or memorabilia that describes who they are as a person and the course of their life. This could be a special photograph, piece of music, ticket or anything that helps us understand more about this person and where they have come from. If the actual item is too special to use for the art piece, a photo copy can be made of it. On the other hand, this could be a way of preserving the important item rather than having it stored in a drawer or other place less visible. Using a mixed media approach, the client can begin by gluing down the significant item at the center of their piece. Next they can surround it colored tissue paper and other collage materials leaving portions of it exposed or not. Finally a thick coating of decoupage glue can be applied to seal the piece.

Description: Values Exploration

Supplies: Pencil, Eraser, Watercolor Pencils, Watercolor Brushes, Watercolor Paper, Water Cup, Paper Towels, Circle to Trace, and Scissors

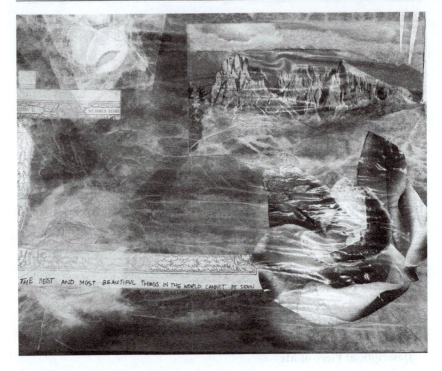

Figure 18.2 Piece of Me Mixed Media Technique.
Source: Photograph and artwork by the author.

Directions: "Values may be described as fundamental attitudes guiding our mental processes and behavior" (Vyskocilova et al., 2015). Values clarification is a subfield in mental health which is linked to Positive Psychology, Cognitive Behavioral Therapy, and Acceptance and Commitment Therapy. Values exploration is an important tool in understanding who were are, where we have come from, and what we feel is most important in life. It can be helpful for understanding others as well. For this art therapy directive, I usually provide the client with a list of possible values as a starting point. I like to use Christopher Peterson and Martin Seligman's (2004) list of values from their seminal book *Character Strengths and Virtues: A Handbook and Classification* because I find their list not too overwhelming yet also encompasses a good amount of options for clients to explore. Once the client has spent time thinking about and exploring these different values, ask them to think about the amount of importance they each hold to them. They can create a mandala using colors and images to represent the different values and how much space they take up in their lives. It can be really powerful in a group to explore the different group members differences and similarities.

Reference List

Jackson, L. (2020). *Cultural humility in art therapy: Applications for practice, research, social justice, self-care, and pedagogy*. London: Jessica Kingsley Publishers.

Peterson, C., & Seligman, M. (2004). *Character strengths and virtues: A handbook and classification*. Washington DC: American Psychological Association and Oxford: Oxford University Press.

Tervalon, M. (2015). *Cultural humility training*. San Mateo, CA: County of San Mateo. [training].

Vyskocilova, J., Prasko, J., Ociskova, M., Sedlackova, Z., & Mozny, P. (2015). Values and values work in cognitive behavioral therapy. *Activitas Nervosa Superior Rediviva*, *57*(1–2), 40–48. doi: 10.1016/j.eurpsy.2016.01.1660.

Chapter 19

Older Adults and Dementia

Older adults, particularly those suffering from dementia and other forms of memory loss, are probably one of the most common populations that art therapists may work with. Art therapy is frequently offered in memory care and assisted living facilities. I was fortunate to work on the geriatric unit at NY Presbyterian Hospital, where I gained experience working with this population and seeing the effectiveness of art therapy on memory. There is more art therapy research in this area than in most other subfields, and it has been proven as an effective way to engage with these clients when they often seem disconnected and isolated. Miller and Johansson (2016) confirm that painting specifically as a medium is helpful because "people with AD have a preserved capability to paint... even those in the later stages of the disease" also "that an artistic development is possible and that painting can be used as an appreciated and beneficial activity for people with AD." Examples of this can be seen in a movie I regularly show in the academic course I teach called *I Remember Better When I Paint* (Ellena, E., & Huebner, 2016). Below are a few art therapy directives for working with older adults using painting as well as other mediums.

Description: Clay Coil Pot

Supplies: Air Dry Clay or Traditional Clay (if a kiln is available), Clay Tools, and Water Cup

Directions: While this directive does not particularly focus on the memory, clay work is useful for older adults who may have motor skills deterioration. I have found from working with older adults without memory impairment, which is important to note, that giving a lot of direction is helpful. However for those suffering from memory impairment working abstractly or with fewer instructions seems more constructive. Creating a simple coil pot is attainable, useful, and excellent for motor skills. Begin by wedging or warming up the clay to get out air bubbles; this is also an added beneficial exercise for the hands of older adults. Next, clients roll small portions of the clay into long

DOI: 10.4324/9781003413363-19

cylindrical strips. The base of the coil pot is a spiral and the walls are formed on the perimeter by spiraling on the outer edge of the base. Be sure to score and slip the coils when joining them together. Lastly, clients can smooth out the coils with their fingers or the clay tools and water.

Description: Doll Making

Supplies: Fabric (or Cotton Socks), Cotton Stuffing, Dried Lavender, Needle, Thread, Scissors, Fabric Markers, Liquid Glue, and other Fiber Art Embellishments

Directions: Sensory and self-soothing projects are a supportive tool for those with memory loss since it can illicit anxiety and some times even anger. Creating a doll or other sensory item can be helpful for providing comfort and reducing anxiety. Similar to the eye pillow directive, dried lavender could be added to the interior stuffing to offer an additional relaxing sensory experience. There are numerous patterns online that the art therapist could refer to for this project which can vary in difficulty based on the client's ability. I have also used a cotton sock for a simpler version. Begin with a plain child's sock or small ankle sock. Then stuff it with cotton stuffing. Using a needle and thread close up the opening to the sock by sewing it shut. Next create legs by stitching down the center toward the bottom from about half way down the sock. Similarly, you can stitch arms by sewing down the sides of the sock body. Lastly, use the thread to tie around the top portion of the sock creating a head. Fabric can be added for clothing by sewing or gluing. Likewise facial details can be added with fabric, markers, or embroidery techniques.

Contraindicated: This project could be considered infantile to some older clients. Additionally, sewing can be challenging for some with memory impairment or fine motor issues. Lastly as mentioned previously, the use of essential oils or lavender can be an overwhelming aroma for those who have a sensitivity to it.

Description: Favorite Tunes

Supplies: Watercolor Paints, Watercolor Brushes, Water Cup, Watercolor Paper, Paper Towels, Music Application and Device for Playing

Directions: Music therapy is a valuable modality for memory care clients, but even simply listening to familiar music is a powerful tool for connecting with those affected by Alzheimer's Disease and dementia. Ask clients to select a favorite song from their past. If this is not possible because the client is non-verbal, select an assortment of music from the general time period when the client grew up. Provide clients with watercolors and let them create abstractly

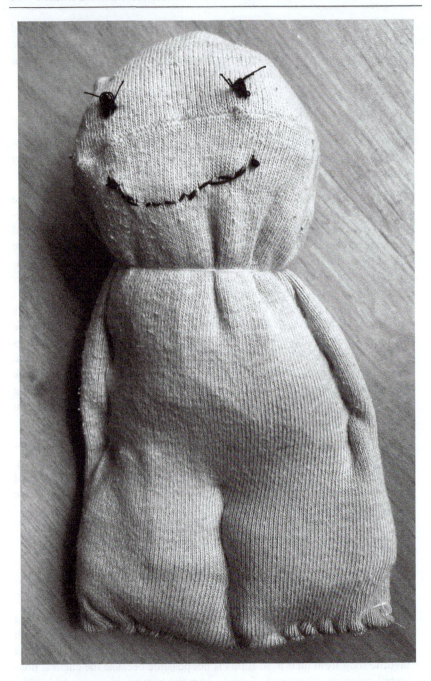

Figure 19.1 Simple Sock Doll Making.

Source: Photograph and artwork by the author.

or realistically while they listen. Watercolor is an easy to use medium with a lot of freedom and flow which is soothing with this population.

Further Reading: For more information on music and memory, I suggest Oliver Sacks' legendary *Musicophilia: Tales of Music and the Brain* (2007).

Description: Velvet Coloring Pages

Supplies: Velvet Coloring Pages, and Washable Markers

Directions: Seemingly very simple, velvet textured coloring pages are useful for those clients with declining vision, tremors, or other mobility challenges that may come with older age. We have used these velvet coloring pages in my art therapy work at acute care hospital settings when working with older adults. I noticed the patients seemed to find them satisfying both because of the sensory soothing nature but also because they were proud of their completed work. These can be purchased online or at arts and crafts supply stores. The textured velvet boundary built into the drawing can help contain the work of the patient making it easier for them to feel confident in their art work while simultaneously providing motor skills practice.

Reference List

Ellena, E., & Huebner, B. (2016). *I remember better when I paint.* Montreuil, France: French Connection Films Hilgos Foundation.

Miller, E., & Johansson, B. (2016). Capability to paint and Alzheimer's disease. *Sage Journals. January-March 2016,* 1–13. doi: 10.1177/2158244016631799.

Sacks, O. (2007). *Musicophilia: Tales of music and the brain.* New York, NY: Vintage Books.

Chapter 20

Personality Disorders

One's personality is the makeup of our unique characteristics, our way of interacting in the world, and our way of thinking, feeling, and behaving. Personality Disorders are a large group of maladaptive behavior patterns that have made interacting in the world and with others difficult. Some Personality Disorders can be genetic but largely our personalities are shaped by our environment and how we grew up. In particular, a Personality Disorder can develop if a person's childhood and adolescent environment was chaotic, violent, and/or neglectful. The Personality Disorders are grouped into three different subcategories or clusters. The main Personality Disorders identified in the fifth edition of the *Diagnostic and Statistical Manual of Mental Disorders* (American Psychiatric Association, 2013) are Paranoid Personality Disorder, Schizoid Personality Disorder, Schizotypal Personality Disorder, Antisocial Personality Disorder, Borderline Personality Disorder, Histrionic Personality Disorder, Narcissistic Personality Disorder, Avoidant Personality Disorder, Dependent Personality Disorder, and Obsessive-Compulsive Personality Disorder. However, treatment for most Personality Disorders is effective and will mainly focus on behavioral therapies rather than psychopharmaceuticals. Though many times Personality Disorders can co-occur with other mental health struggles and diagnoses. During the time when I worked at New York Presbyterian, they offered a mental health unit specifically dedicated to working with people who have Personality Disorders and the clinicians were exceptionally skilled. There are numerous residential treatment centers that treat each specific Personality Disorder as well, since often retraining the way we interact after many years of operating in a certain way is challenging. Most often Cognitive Behavioral Therapies and those based similarly, such as Dialectical Behavior Therapy and Acceptance and Commitment Therapy, are the treatment of choice for Personality Disorders and you will see those techniques integrated into the art therapy directives below.

Further Reading: *DBT-Informed Art Therapy: Mindfulness, Cognitive Behavior Therapy, and the Creative Process* by Susan M. Clark (2016).

DOI: 10.4324/9781003413363-20

Description: Decorative Diary Cards

Supplies: 3 × 5 or 4 × 6 Index Cards, Pencil, Eraser, Colored Pencils, and Fine Point Markers

Directions: As referred to in earlier chapters, Dialectical Behavior Therapy is the treatment of choice for many Personality Disorders. One of the techniques used frequently in Dialectical Behavior Therapy are called Diary Cards. Diary Cards are a way for clients to track if they have used their Dialectical Behavior Therapy skills during times of distress or strong emotions. This can

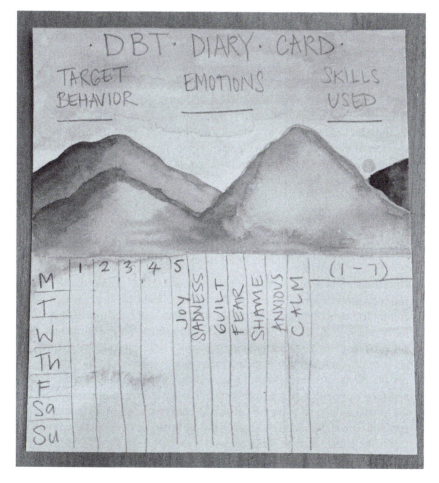

Figure 20.1 Decorative Diary Card.

Source: Photograph and artwork by the author.

in turn help the client decipher which specific Dialectical Behavior Therapy technique was most effective for them. While not traditional art, clients could take their time creating their own personalized Diary Cards in a more creative and perhaps aesthetically pleasing way. If the client enjoys the cards they have created, maybe they will remember and want to use them more often.

Description: Distress Tolerance

Supplies: Drawing Paper, Pencil, Eraser, Colored Pencil, and Laminating Equipment

Directions: The developer of Dialectical Behavior Therapy skills Marsha Linehan (2014) describes distress tolerance as "a person's ability to manage an emotional incident without feeling overwhelmed." This is an important skill for everyone to learn. It requires practice when not in distress so that these skills can be accessed during highly emotional times. For this art therapy directive, ask clients to create a list of their best and most affective distress tolerance skills. Examples may include: self soothing, distractions, removing yourself, or splashing your face with cold water. Rather than make a list, create drawings or symbols of these techniques. As a way to keep the list accessible, laminate the drawing so that it can be preserved and kept in a spot easy for the client to see like on a dresser, desk, or the refrigerator.

Description: Interpersonal Comic

Supplies: Drawing Paper, Pre-printed Blank Comic Strips, Pencil, Eraser, Colored Pencil, Pens, and Fine Point Black Marker

Directions: Struggling with interpersonal skills is a characteristic that is common with various Personality Disorders. Clients can begin with a blank comic strip either pre-printed from the art therapist or hand drawn to customize themselves. Ask the client to think of a recent or on-going interpersonal situation that they have been struggling with. The client can portray the typical scenario on the comic strip and their usual response to this. Next the client and therapist can brainstorm a second way of responding to the situation and they can draw a second version of the comic as a comparison. Perhaps the client could even come up with additional responses to the interpersonal scenario as well. Some of these may also be humorous over exaggerations or things the client might never even do.

Description: Wise Mind

Supplies: Pencil, Eraser, Watercolor Pencils, Watercolor Brushes, Watercolor Paper, Water Cup, and Paper Towels

Directions: In Dialectical Behavior Therapy one of the main themes of the work is the use of the 'Wise Mind' and walking the middle path. Begin this session with psycho education around this concept. Have the client draw two circles overlapping in the middle, in the style of a Venn diagram. One of the circles is the 'Emotional Mind' and the other is the 'Rational Mind' with the 'Wise Mind' in the middle overlapping portion. Ask the client to use water-color to make the 'Wise Mind' a certain color that expresses characteristics of that state of mind. Then ask the client come up with an alternative color to express the characteristics of the 'Rational Mind.' Lastly the combined colors can be created and put into the 'Wise Mind' portion which is of course a blending of the two minds.

Reference List

American Psychiatric Association. (2013). *Diagnostic and statistical manual of mental disorders* (5th ed.). Arlington, TX: American Psychiatric Association.

Clark, S. (2016). *DBT-informed art therapy: Mindfulness, cognitive behavior therapy, and the creative process*. London: Jessica Kingsley Publishers.

Chapter 21

Pregnancy, Infertility, and Women's Health

Women's health, pregnancy, and loss are a niche within the field of mental health that often doesn't get recognized and supported enough, particularly because of the shame or embarrassment that may sometimes come along with it. Art therapy in a group format is especially helpful with this population for just that reason. Many times, issues too difficult to discuss are more easily explored through art making, as we well know being art therapists. Additionally, the beauty of group therapy is the understanding that you are not alone in what you are going through. Art therapy groups could explore new motherhood and postpartum blues, or more severe mood disorders. Another common theme that is often covered in support groups is pregnancy loss and infertility. I hope these women's health support groups become more available, especially incorporating the use of art therapy and below are some techniques that may apply.

Further Reading: An underrepresented area in the field of psychology in general and certainly in art therapy, Nora Swan-Foster's edited collection titled *Art Therapy and Childbearing Issues* (2020) has some important work on the topics of pregnancy, loss, and other women's issues.

Description: Clay Imprint

Supplies: White Air Dry Clay (Model Magic® is my preference for this project), Markers, and Clay Tools

Directions: Begin by warming up the clay. Add washable marker to it and wedge it until a desired color is formed, repeating this as needed until the chosen shade is reached. Next, roll the clay out flat with a sculpting tool or I often just use the round marker that we were using for adding color. Clients can then create their own shape or use something round to trace and cut out as a base. Depending on the specific theme of the group, clients can select something significant to imprint into the clay. Examples could include: important initials, memorabilia, words of support, or even finger prints. Lastly, use a clay tool or pencil to create a small hole in the top. These imprints could be hung somewhere in the house or made into jewelry.

DOI: 10.4324/9781003413363-21

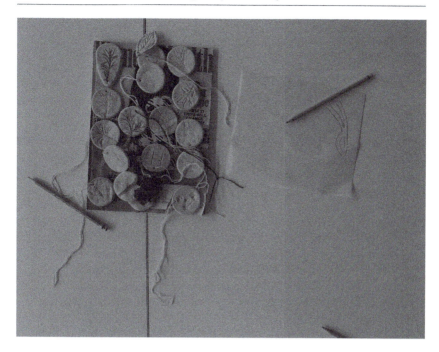

Figure 21.1 Clay Imprints.

Source: Photograph by the author.

Description: Growth Printmaking Series

Supplies: Styrofoam for Printmaking, Ballpoint Pen, Printmaking Ink, Disposable Paint Palette, Brayer, and Mixed Media Paper

Directions: For this art therapy directive, ask clients to think of something in nature during the growing process. This could be an animal, flower, fruit, or other fauna. Clients can create a practice sketch of their creation including at least three images in the growth process. Next, clients draw these images onto three separate Styrofoam sheets using a ball point pen. These Styrofoam sheets can be purchased online or at art supply stores. On a tight budget I have used Styrofoam trays from the grocery store, but they can often be too thick making it difficult to get detail. Once the drawings are completed, clients can choose to print them one on top of another or in a row. Spread printing ink on a palette or plate and use the brayer to collect the ink and roll it onto the Styrofoam image before printing it onto paper.

Note: It is important to let clients know that the image will be printed backward. If it is meaningful that the image be printed in a certain direction, I recommend making the sketch onto tracing paper which can then be flipped before tracing it with the pen onto the Styrofoam. I also suggest to clients that they avoid using words since it can be difficult because of this same reason.

Description: Hygge

Supplies: Drawing Paper, Chalk Pastel, Charcoal Sticks, Blending Sticks, Oil pastels or Colored Pencil

Directions: I have been writing this book from Norway while on sabbatical and "hygge" is a comforting Scandinavian tradition here that I will take with me back home. It was born out of the long, dark winters. While waiting for news about pregnancy, grieving a loss, or other fertility related stressors, we need to be gentle on ourselves. This is the essence of the Scandinavian tradition of surrounding yourself or participating in activities which promote a sense of calm and contentment. Begin the session by focusing on the importance of the environment as a place of comfort. A few example of this could be: lighting a candle, aromatherapy, comfortable seating, and cozy blankets. Next ask the client to think of things that bring them comfort and create images to represent this. Often the simple act of making the art and setting up the environment is a satisfying example of hygge, but it is nice to think of other easy ways to incorporate this tradition for when needed.

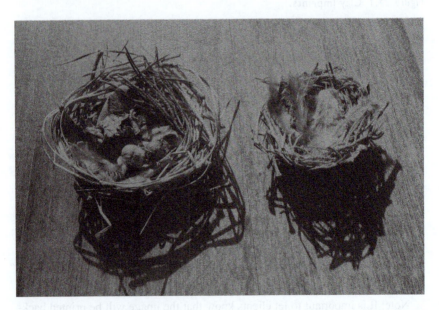

Figure 21.2 Nest Examples.

Source: Photograph and artwork by the author.

Description: Nest

Supplies: Natural Materials for Building the Nest (i.e.- small twigs, recycled paper, raffia), Disposable Bowl, Spray Adhesive, and Additional Materials for Inside the Nest

Directions: For this art therapy directive, clients can build a nest from natural materials. I used pine needles collected from my yard since we live in a wooded area. Begin by sculpting the shape of the nest on top of a small disposable paper or plastic bowl, shaping the fibers and adding adhesive as you go to secure them. Clients can use any sort of other sculpted or natural materials placed into their nest or leave it simply as a nest depending on the particular work the client is focusing on with the art therapist. Perhaps the client wants to focus more on nest building rather than what goes into it or vice versa.

Reference List

Swan-Foster, N. (2020). *Art therapy and childbearing issues*. New York, NY: Routledge.

Chapter 22

Psychotic Disorders

One of the most challenging populations to work with are those affected by psychosis due to Schizophrenia, Schizoaffective Disorder, or other severe mental illnesses. While I worked at New York Presbyterian, I had the opportunity to provide art therapy on the various mental health units, one of them being dedicated to Psychotic Disorders. It can be difficult to work in groups with this population due to the varying differences in ability and acuity from person to person. Generally speaking, sensory-related and soothing activities prove valuable to these types of patients. Depending on the severity of the patients, the art therapist needs to be mindful of the material choices because of safety concerns and facility rules. Below are a few art therapy directives I have found beneficial for this type of patient.

Description: Grounding with the Five Senses

Supplies: 5 sheets of 8.5 × 11 Drawing Paper (or one larger sheet divided into sections), Pencil, Eraser, Markers or Colored Pencils

Directions: While this is a traditional grounding technique often used for anxiety, PTSD and panic attacks, I have found it can be helpful also with patients who struggle to stay in the present. Patients can work on five separate sheets of paper or with one large piece divided into sections. Begin with psycho education about the use of the five senses as a grounding technique. If necessary, patients can write down on their paper the five senses as a reminder. Ask patients to draw something they can identify in the room or nearby that correlates to each of the five senses.

Description: Drawing to Music

Supplies: Large Sheets of Drawing Paper, Chalk Pastel, Washable Markers, Oil Pastel, Application to Play Music, Device and Speaker to Play Music

DOI: 10.4324/9781003413363-22

Directions: This is a creative arts directive that was utilized at New York Presbyterian on the Psychotic Disorders unit. Seemingly very simple, it was generally a group activity the patients all looked forward to. Listening to music
while making art can comfort most people while engaging them at the same
time. This desired level of alert yet calm is challenging to achieve with this
population when medications are often being adjusted and patients may be experiencing side effects. Ask patients to each select a song while they make art
with minimal directions. The art therapist plays disc jockey to the patient's
requests that can vary from uplifting to more meaningful serious selections.
Lastly patients can process their art work and share if there are any connections
to the music.

Description: Mono Printing

Supplies: Small Plexi-Glass Sheets (roughly 8 x 10), Printmaking Ink, Printmaking Brayer, Disposable Paint Palettes, Paint Brushes, Water Cup, Paper
Towels, and Mixed Media Paper, Colored Pencil, Fine Point Markers, Watercolor Pencils, and Watercolor Brushes

Directions: The beauty of this printmaking technique is that it is comprised
of abstract shapes and colors rather than anything realistic. Begin by explaining to patients that this exercise is just about putting down colors and shapes
that they find attractive and interesting. Have the patient apply printing ink
colors onto the disposable palette or directly onto the plexiglass. If applying
it directly onto the plexiglass, use smaller amounts. However the printing
ink does dry quickly so it is important to move relatively swiftly. Paint the
ink onto the plexi-glass in abstract shapes and colors until a desired design is
completed. Then make the print by pressing the mixed media paper on top of
the plexi-glass and follow with a brayer making sure to apply pressure to all
areas. Depending on how much ink was applied, often multiple prints can be
made from the same plexi-glass with varying gradations of colors. Another
different print can also be made by not rinsing off the original painted design
and then applying another right on top.

Variation: If the group or session is ongoing and the client and art therapist
have at least two sessions together, there is a second step that could be incorporated into this mono printing technique. Once dried, the patient can go back
into the print with color penciled, fine point markers, or watercolors to add
supplementary designs or words.

Description: Watercolor Abstract

Supplies: Watercolor Paints, Watercolor Brushes, Watercolor Paper, Water
Cup, and Paper Towels

Directions: Watercolor as a medium can be very soothing, particularly when working abstractly. Show patients some basic watercolor techniques especially wet-on-wet for this exercise. Be sure to use watercolor paper for this exercise or it will not be successful. Apply a large amount of water to the paper and have patients explore how the paint interacts and moves on the watery surface.

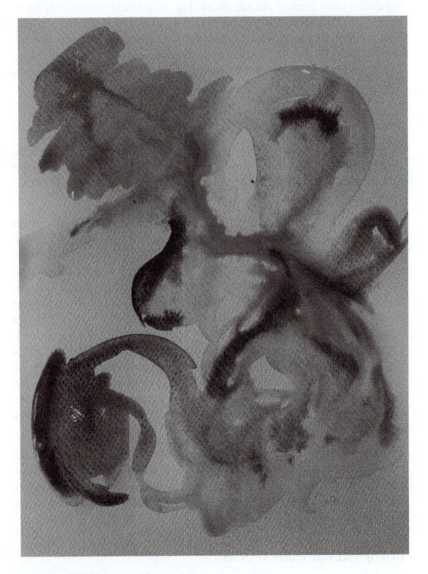

Figure 22.1 Watercolor Abstract.

Source: Photograph and artwork by the author.

Chapter 23

Self-Esteem

The way we feel about ourselves can affect our entire world. Poor self-esteem can limit our friendships, intimate relationships, and career aspirations, and prevent clients from progressing in life. Self-esteem can be influenced by childhood experiences, unhealthy relationships, unfortunate life events, unrealistic societal pressures, and social media. Self-esteem can also affect mood and may eventually lead to prolonged depression and anxiety. Most people have experienced moments in their lives when they do not feel their best or may question their abilities, and therefore, working in this area is beneficial to so many of us and throughout the life span. However, it is more common to see lower self-esteem generally in women, adolescents, and young adults. One beautiful part of art therapy is the sense of pride we often see when our clients successfully complete a project. While not always the focus of art therapy though when a client makes an art piece that they feel is successful or pleasing to the eye, it is powerful. Taking that a step further, at some of the in-patient hospitals and treatment centers I have worked at, we held annual art exhibits. It was during these art shows that I saw patient's pride and esteem blossom. It is important to note that clients need to be made aware ahead of art making that they have the option to exhibit their artwork. This will of course put a different spin on their artwork, but it is therapeutic in a different sense. The power of sharing our art in a group is meaningful and is an added self-esteem boost to the process of art making alone. Below are a few art therapy directives that may be helpful in working on increasing self-esteem through their focus on affirmations and positive sense of self.

Description: Affirmation Word

Supplies: Watercolor Paints, Watercolor Paper (cut into a rectangular shape), Watercolor Brushes, Pencil, Eraser, Paper Towels, and Water Cup

Directions: For this directive, ask clients to think of an affirmation word that they feel will be a helpful reminder to themselves regarding their self-esteem. The client may not even believe this word at the time of creation, but this is something

DOI: 10.4324/9781003413363-23

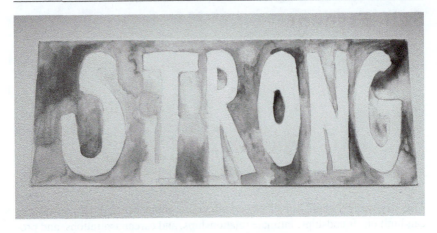

Figure 23.1 Affirmation Word Watercolor.

Source: Photograph and artwork by the author.

they would like to embody eventually. Begin with a rectangular piece of watercolor paper. To get the spacing correct on the letters, I suggest to clients that they lightly write small letters in pencil above where the larger block letters will go. Otherwise, clients could run out of space as they write the block letters which could frustrate them. I then have clients either watercolor inside the letters leaving the outside white or watercolor the outside and leave the letters white. The point is for the word to be a bold reminder to the client of their worth.

Description: Affirmation Journal

Supplies: 12 × 18 Drawing Paper, Pencil, Eraser, Scissors, Metal Spoon, Embroidery Floss, Awl Tool, and Needle

Directions: Daily affirmations are a practice that can benefit clients working on self-esteem. Rather than just verbalizing them, clients can enter them into a handmade journal on a daily basis to reflect back on and try to initiate new daily affirmations. There are a variety of ways to make your own journal or booklet and below I have described two different techniques. The first book is simpler and uses only paper and scissors, while the second version incorporates a sewn binding. I learned these bookmaking techniques in my graduate art education program at Lesley University.

Steps: Simple Folded Book

- As I mentioned with origami, I like to use cardinal directions when explaining these folding steps as well.

- Begin with the 12 × 18 paper laying horizontally in front of you.
- Next fold the top half (North) to meet the bottom half (South).
- Then fold the West side to meet the East side.
- Next repeat that two more times until you have a small rectangle.
- Unfold the paper completely and then fold the West side to meet the East side again.
- Take your scissors and cut from the West side into the center just one section length.
- Again unfold the paper completely and there should be a slit in the center taking up the two middle sections.
- Fold the top North side down to meet the bottom South side and then push the edges together until you see a three dimensional box form in the center. Continue to push it until it becomes flat.
- Lastly fold it all together into a booklet shape creasing all the folds sharply using a metal spoon. You should now have a small six page book.

Steps: Bound Book

- Start by deciding of the number of interior pages, you would like for this book.
- Use one sheet of colored construction paper for the cover and several sheets of plain white computer paper for the interior pages. Note, you will have double the original amount.
- Using 8 × 11.5 plain printer paper fold them in half. Use a metal spoon to crease the centerfold deeply.
- Then create four or six spots down the center seam where you will make holes to create the binding. Note, this needs to be an even number though.
- It is helpful to mark these with pencil first. Then using an awl tool, poke the holes in all these predetermined locations.
- Next using the embroidery floss, loop it through two of the holes next to each other with the ends dangling outward. Do the same for the other additional holes.
- Lastly a double knot or bow can be tied on the exterior to secure the embroidery floss. It can be interesting to use multiple colors of embroidery floss for this decorative binding.

Description: Assertiveness Training

Supplies: 12 × 18 Drawing Paper, Pencil, Eraser, Markers, Colored Pencils, or Pens

Directions: Provide psycho education on the four main types communication styles. These are Passive, Passive Aggressive, Assertive, Aggressive. Have clients create a spectrum line of these communication styles. They could create symbols or words to mark these communication styles along the spectrum line. Next have clients draw themselves and others in different scenarios or varying relationships along the spectrum. Clients should consider in which relationships or scenarios they use assertiveness as compared to the alternative communication styles.

Description: Gift to Yourself

Supplies: Small Paper Mache Craft Boxes (size 3" L × 3" W × 1-1/2" H), Magazines, Scissors, Glue Sticks, Decoupage Glue and Brush (Mod Podge® is my preference for this project), Permanent Markers, Colored Pencils, or Oil Pastels

Directions: Ask clients to think about a gift they would like to give themselves. Steer clients away from material goods and focus instead on intangible themes. For clients that often put themselves last, they may enjoy things like: time to themselves, better boundaries, or rekindling old friendships. Clients can decorate the outside of the box to look like a gift or anything they find aesthetically pleasing with collage or other two-dimensional materials. Then on the inside, have clients use collage as a medium to represent their particular gift or as many as they feel are important. Lastly, use a coating of the decoupage glue to seal the collage down and create a smooth shiny protective outer layer on the box.

Chapter 24

Spirituality

Leonardo da Vinci famously said, "Where the spirit does not work with the hand, there is no art." Art and spirituality merge together magnificently. Spirituality is different for each person, but an exploration into the meaning of why we are here on the planet may likely come up in sessions. Some clients may be confident in their spirituality, especially if they have endured a health scare, loss, or other traumatic life experience. While other clients may be looking at their spirituality from a more existential point of view or as they come of age. Additionally, spirituality is a part of the Alcoholics Anonymous program, and for our clients working on sobriety, they may refer to it as a higher power. Spirituality can encompass time in nature, connecting with one's heritage, yoga, music, art making, or traditional organized religions. I have witnessed the spiritual transcendence of the art making process in individual sessions as well as in art therapy groups when the art makes us connect to something larger than just ourselves. For clients trying to connect and understand their own spirituality, art making can be a helpful tool, and below are a few art therapy directives that may facilitate that.

Further Reading: For a deeper dive into art therapy and spirituality, I recommend *Spirituality and Art Therapy: Living the Connection*, edited by Mimi Farrelly-Hansen (2001).

Description: Awe

Supplies: Drawing Paper, Pencil, Eraser, Colored Pencil, Chalk Pastel, Charcoal Sticks and Blending Stick

Directions: Awe is a complicated feeling that has recently gained interest in the field of psychology. While hard to describe, most people can think of a time when they felt awe. It is a mix of amazement and fear both positive and negative emotions. Most commonly people think of it as when they have a goosebump sensation. The benefit of the feeling of awe is that it can make us feel connected to something much bigger than just ourselves which can in turn help clients gain perspective, resilience, and potential happiness. For this art therapy directive, ask clients to think of a time in their lives when they

DOI: 10.4324/9781003413363-24

may have experienced awe. They can recreate the experience using two dimensional or three dimensional materials, but my preference for this directive would be chalk pastel because of its ethereal quality.

Description: Heart and Soul

Supplies: Mixed Media Paper, Black Permanent Marker, Watercolor Paints, Watercolor Brushes, Water Cup, and Paper Towel

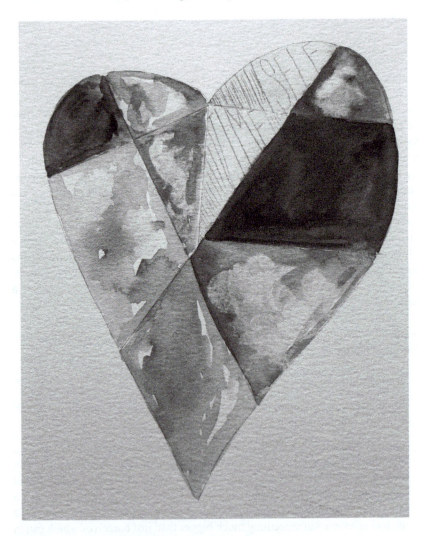

Figure 24.1 Heart and Soul Watercolor.

Source: Photograph and artwork by the author.

Directions: Spiritual wellness is the checking in on our connection with our own spirituality. In this directive, clients can explore this idea further by looking at where in their lives they connect spiritually and where they might like to develop it further. Beginning with watercolor paper, have clients create a large heart shape as the boundary for the piece. Ask clients to think about the various ways in which they may connect with their own spirituality. They can chose colors to represent their different spiritual practices in their life (i.e. meditation, volunteering, or church). They can also look at the amount of space they each take up and maybe leave areas still open based on their current spiritual wellness.

Description: Soul Collage®

Supplies: Card Stock or Mat Board cut into 5x8 Rectangles, Magazines, Scissors, Glue Sticks, Decoupage Glue and Brush (Mod Podge® is my preference for this project)

Note: This art therapy modality needs several sessions to be completed.

Directions: Soul Collage® is a registered trademarked collage technique often led by trained facilitators originally created by psychologist Seena Frost. Additional training is available for art therapists interested in taking a deeper dive into this specialized technique. The process is lengthy and would involve numerous sessions for your client or group. The process begins by making a deck of cards using collage as the medium. Next participants use a specific phrase to embody the card's perspective "I am one who..." and to give it a title. There are various types of sets a participant could create and therefor I would suggest exploring further the Soul Collage® web site or their books as a way to learn more if interested. Lastly participants would use their own deck to pull from for spiritual guidance in times of need or with life questions.

Description: Your Creation Story

Supplies: Drawing Paper, Pencil, Eraser, Colored Pencil, Marker, Oil Pastel, or Chalk Pastel

Directions: This art therapy directive was designed in collaboration with one of my colleagues at the William & Mary Wellness Center who is a chaplain when we co-facilitated a group on art and spirituality for the students. Ask clients to think of their own life history as well as that of their relatives or ancestors. Clients can create images that tell this story using two-dimensional materials. This can be the client's personal life story or a bigger picture exploration of their family lineage.

Reference List

Farrelly-Hansen, M. (Ed.). (2001). *Spirituality and art therapy: Living the connection.* London: Jessica Kingsley Publishers.

Frost, S.B. Soul Collage. (2023). *Soul Collage.* Retrieved from https://soulcollage.com.

Chapter 25

Substance Abuse and Addiction

When working with patients and clients struggling with addiction, art therapy can be a helpful tool for people to reflect on their past and think about the changes they would like to make for their future. Sometimes clients may also have co-occurring mental health diagnoses. However, for this section, I will focus solely on substance abuse recovery work. One of the gold standards for the treatment of addictions is of course utilizing the step work in Alcoholics or Narcotics Anonymous. Self-Management and Recovery Training, also known as S.M.A.R.T., is another support group and program that many have found life-saving. In my experience working on in-patient mental health units, I have also noticed various cognitive-behavioral therapy techniques to be highly effective. You will find some of these modalities incorporated into the art therapy directives in this section.

Further Reading: For a more in-depth exploration on the topic of substance abuse and addiction treatment through art therapy, I recommend *Art Therapy and Substance Abuse* by Libby Schmanke (2017).

Description: Cognitive Distortions

Supplies: Drawing Paper, Pencil, Eraser, Colored Pencils, Markers, Pens, Chalk Pastel, or Oil Pastel

Directions: Begin by providing psycho education about cognitive distortions, a well-known cognitive behavioral therapy model (Positive Psychology, 2023). I usually print out a handout from online with the main cognitive distortions and their definitions to give to the client as well. I really like the Cognitive Distortions handout by PositivePsychology.com for this. After talking about the main 15 different cognitive distortions, ask clients to think about one they may use in their life, especially as it relates to their addiction. Once clients have decided on a cognitive distortion to focus on, ask them to think about how it might go alternatively. For example, using the cognitive distortion "blaming." If the client

DOI: 10.4324/9781003413363-25

believes they drink too much because their work is too stressful. Perhaps they could to try envision and create an image not using "blame" in their recovery.

Description: Higher Power

Supplies: Air Dry Clay, Clay Tools, Water Cup, Mixed Media Paper, Pencil, Eraser, Watercolor Paint, Acrylic Paint, Paint Brushes, Paint Palette, and Paper Towels

Directions: This directive is for clients who are working the Twelve Steps in Alcoholics or Narcotics Anonymous. Ask clients to reflect on their relationship with their higher power as it relates to their recovery. For this art therapy directive, clients can use two or three dimensional materials, air dry clay could be another medium suggestion, but I leave it up to the client to decide. Ask the client to create two main figures, the self and their higher power, and how they relate along with their proximity to one another.

Description: Safe Haven

Supplies: Plaster Cloth Strips, Bowl of Warm Water, Rubber Balloons, Acrylic Paint, Paint Palette, Paint Brushes, and Clear Plastic String

Note: This art therapy directive needs to be completed in two separate sessions due to drying time of the plaster.

Directions: Going through recovery can be a challenging and scary process. Ask clients to think about what their safe haven might look like or encompass within it. This could be a place with things they find centering in times of distress or when they feel triggered. Maybe these items are more concrete like certain people and soothing objects or perhaps they are more abstract like ideals like security or a peaceful mind. I learned this art technique from Ideas Magazine in the March 2014 issue and turned it into this art therapy directive. Begin by having clients blow up a rubber balloon approximately the size of a grapefruit. Next lay the wet plaster strips onto the balloon one at a time smoothing out the small holes in the plaster. Generally, I recommend two complete layers of plaster all over the balloon except for the center opening. This plaster layer will need to harden overnight and then the balloon can be popped and removed. Next clients can paint the outside of the haven as they desire, maybe using some protective images. Then they can paint the inside of the haven with their safety and comfort themes. Lastly, clients can make a pin hole at the top and thread through string for hanging.

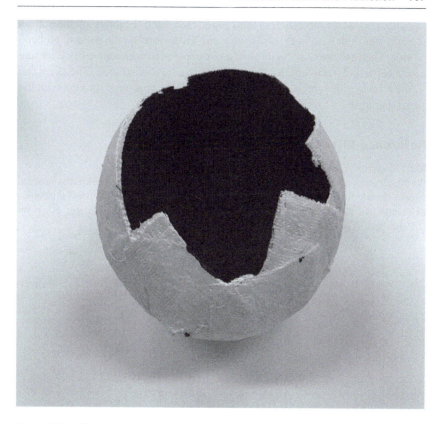

Figure 25.1 Plaster Safe Haven (in Progress).

Source: Photograph by Lindsay Heck and artwork by the author.

Description: Thoughts Feelings Behaviors

Supplies: Drawing Paper, Pencil, Eraser, Markers, Colored Pencils or Crayons

Directions: The CBT model of the Thoughts, Feelings, Behavior Triangle has been a gold standard for behavior change since its inception by psychologist Aaron Beck. Beck was one of the pioneers of Cognitive Behavioral Therapy. The head psychiatrist on the adolescent hospital unit where I worked for years operated from a cognitive behavioral framework. He was not only a kind and gentle person, but an excellent teacher who has influenced my own approaches to art therapy. Cognitive Behavioral Therapy is a useful methodology when working with clients struggling with addiction and substance abuse because it can help alter mal-adaptive behavior patterns and reframe thinking. Begin with basic psycho education around Cognitive Behavioral theory and the Thoughts, Feelings, Behaviors Triangle. Have the client write the word

'Thoughts' at the top center of their paper, then write 'Feelings' on the bottom right hand side, and lastly write the word 'Behaviors' on the bottom left hand side. Then ask the client to think of an example of a maladaptive behavior that relates to their recovery that they could utilize for this exercise. The client can draw images or symbols to represent these while working it through with the art therapist.

Reference List

Ideas Magazine. (2014, March). *Paper Mache Nests*, 27.
PositivePsychology.(2023).*Cognitivedistortions*.Retrievedfromhttps://positivepsychology.
  com/cbt-cognitive-behavioral-therapy-techniques-worksheets/#cognitive-distortions.
Schmanke, L. (2017). *Art therapy and substance abuse*. London: Jessica Kingsley
  Publishers.

Chapter 26

Supervision

As registered and/or board-certified art therapists, we may often provide supervision to other art therapists throughout our careers. Beginning in graduate school, art therapy interns will need on-site supervisors as well as certified art therapy supervisors. Then, as the credentialing process continues, provisional art therapist will need early career supervision as well. Additionally, many registered or board-certified art therapists engage in peer supervision throughout their career life span as well. Supervision can be provided on an individual or group basis. The Art Therapy Credentials Board also offers an advanced certification for supervisors if desired. Some of my most pivotal therapeutic moments have come from supervision work both in my graduate program as well as with peer supervisors at the in-patient hospitals where I have worked. I found it invaluable to work amongst peers at both the Brattleboro Retreat and New York Presbyterian for just this reason. Unfortunately, it can be more rare in our field to work with other creative arts therapists and to be the sole art therapist at a place of work which can feel isolating. It is in those instances that I have sought out peer supervision groups. Below are a few art therapy directives that are particular to art therapy supervision.

Description: Case Reflection

Supplies: Two or Three Dimensional Materials

Directions: Seemingly very simple but often remarkably powerful as art therapists, is to make art in reflection to a particular client or case. For a case that is either challenging or making the art therapist feel unusual feelings, taking time to make art in reflection to this case can provide insight. In my graduate program at Pratt Institute we were encouraged to explore feelings of counter-transference to the client or patient. Counter-transference is natural and understanding it better can help gain awareness into unconscious experiences between the client and therapist which may be a recapitulation of what the client experiences in their own life. Once the supervisee has made a reflection piece, it can be enlightening for the art therapist supervisor to share

DOI: 10.4324/9781003413363-26

their interpretation of the art work and process together personal experiences that may be impacting the case. As art therapists, we need little guidance on materials and therefor for this directive the medium is up to the supervisee.

Description: Chakras

Supplies: Mixed Media Paper, Pencil, Eraser, Colored Pencil, Watercolor Paints, Watercolor Pencils, Watercolor Brushes, Water Cup, and Paper Towels

Directions: Another tool for gaining insight into a challenging client or case can be to connect with ones body to better understand what is going on. While

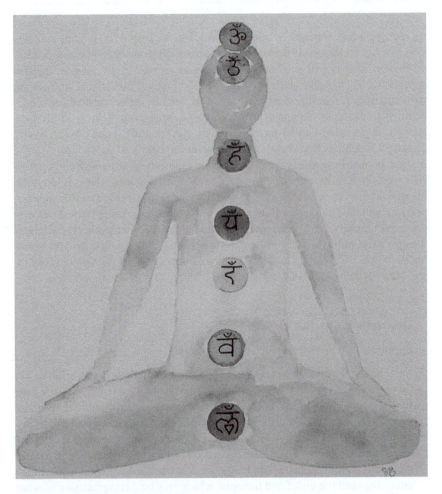

Figure 26.1 Chakras Watercolor Reflection.
Source: Artwork by the author.

yogic and energy practices may not be for everyone, connecting with your body as a tool for deeper understanding is important as creative arts therapists. My graduate program at Pratt Institute integrated dance movement therapy techniques into our studies. I also have graduated from a yoga teacher training which I would also recommend for creative arts therapists. If this is an idea that the art therapy supervisee is interested in, begin by discussing the background of the particular case or work situation that may be troubling them. Ask the supervisee to think about where in the body they feel the situation. It may be helpful to show the supervisee a diagram of the seven chakras which can be printed out from online. Depending on the skill set of the art therapist, they can give education about the different chakras and their meanings or ask the supervisee to study about this as "homework" as it relates to their case in question.

Variation: Rather than having the art therapy supervisee research the particular chakra, they could additionally or alternatively make art about the specific chakra using its coordinating color.

Description: Help for the Helper

Supplies: Drawing Paper Cut into a Circular Shape, Pencil, Eraser, Colored Pencil or Markers

Directions: For those starting out in the field of mental health, some times the work can feel very intense. This may be because it is our first work experience with those in need or also because most internships are often in acute hospital settings. At the beginning of my art therapy career, I remember experiencing burn out and not knowing how to take care of myself. For this art therapy directive, ask the supervisee to create a self-care mandala. This mandala could be abstract or perhaps a more specific and realistic look at their self-care needs. Begin by having the supervisee think about how they care for themselves in relation to their work. Ask them to portray these different self-care skills inside the mandala taking up as much space as they practice them in their own life. Maybe there is room for more self-care skills to be learned in supervision that can later be added to the mandala.

Description: Vision Board

Supplies: Large Piece of Poster Board, Pencil, Eraser, Permanent Markers, Pens, Magazines, Scissors, Glue Sticks, Decoupage Glue and Brush (Mod Podge® is my preference for this project)

Directions: Vision boards are traditionally a technique utilized by life coaches and are useful for goal setting. For this art therapy directive, the focus will be on the career goals of the supervisee. Begin with a large sheet of card stock or poster board and gather materials for collage and mixed media. Ask the supervisee to think of various art therapy career goals. Maybe they want to get certified or specialize in a certain sub specialty in the field or maybe they want to attain board certification status? Maybe the supervisee would like to switch careers within the field or open a private practice? Once the supervisee has set some goals and put them on to the vision board, they can begin to think about the steps it would take to get there for each of the goals. All of the goals and steps to get there can be collaged on to the vision board, written out, or a combination of the two.

Variation: Alternatively supervisees could create this digitally if that is the art therapist's preference since then it could be more readily available if this is something they might consult frequently.

Chapter 27

Termination

Traditionally, termination refers to ending the therapeutic relationship between the therapist and the client. In broader terms, it can also mean when a therapeutic group is ending or when a patient is graduating from a residential treatment program. In my work at the university level, or perhaps in therapeutic schools, this could be the end of the semester. This is a critical stage in the therapeutic process as it represents, in general, how we handle separations, goodbyes, grief, and important milestones. It is best to begin talking about and planning for this in advance with clients and patients so they can mentally prepare for the goodbye. It may be instinctive for some clients and patients to want to "ghost" or even skip the final goodbye, but working through these hard feelings is all part of the work. It can also prompt important discussions about previous goodbyes, deaths, or other relationship endings. Below are a few art therapy directives that are especially applicable to termination.

Description: Gateway

Supplies: Drawing Paper, Scissors, Pencil, Eraser, Colored Pencils, Charcoal Sticks, Blending Stick, Chalk Pastel, or Oil Pastel

Directions: This directive focuses on moving on from the past and looking toward the future. Clients are asked to think of something they are proud of moving on from and what they are looking forward to in the future. Clients then fold their paper into thirds with the edges meeting in the center. They can then choose to create any sort of doorway, gate, or opening on the outside and this may contain images of whatever it is they are moving on from. On the inside of the paper, clients can then create an image or symbol to represent their future hopes and plans.

Description: Goodbye and Hello

Supplies: Watercolor Paper cut into 5 × 8 size, Pencil, Watercolor Paints, Watercolor Brushes, Water Cup, and Paper Towel

DOI: 10.4324/9781003413363-27

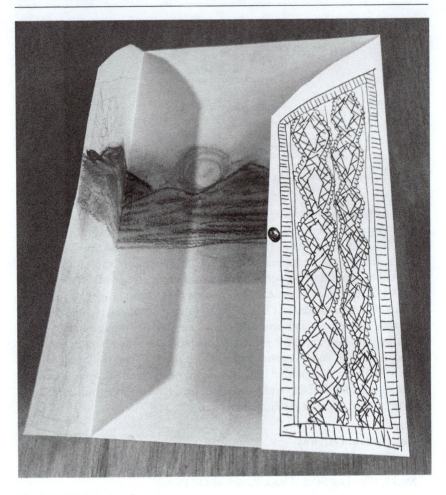

Figure 27.1 Gateway Drawing.

Source: Photograph and artwork by the author.

Directions: Generally, when a client is ready to terminate from therapy, hopefully they have moved past a certain issue or behavior. For this directive, clients can write a letter or I usually have pre-made post card style pieces made out of watercolor paper as another option. Ask the client to think about something they have said goodbye to during your to work together. Inevitably they will have something new in place of that to say hello to. An example of this could be, stopping a maladaptive behavior and replacing it with a healthy coping skill. Clients can use the blank side of the paper to create an image to represent this transformation. On the back the client could write a goodbye and hello message to these behaviors.

Variation: For group termination, participants can do a scaled down version making one for each of their peers. They could create mini-post cards depicting something significant they are proud of the person for or important things they will remember them for.

Description: Rose, Thorn, Bud

Supplies: Origami Paper and Pencil

Directions: This is an activity that I often do with my own family at the end of the day as a verbal check in. I thought of adapting it for a termination art therapy directive by adding the art making process as a transitional object. To mark the end of a therapeutic relationship, ask the client to think about their rose, thorn, and bud of their work in your sessions or therapeutic group together. The rose would be their highlight or something they are proud of. The thorn would be their hardest part of the work together. Lastly, the bud would be something they are looking forward to moving forward. Begin by asking the group members two write these three things on the plain side of their origami paper.

Steps: This origami project uses two different sheets of origami paper. One for the flower and one for the stem.

- Begin with the decorative side of the paper down on the table and the white side facing up.
- Place the paper in the shape of a diamond on the table.
- Again, I like to use cardinal directions when explaining origami steps.
- Take the South point of the paper and bring it to the North Point, making a sharp crease across the middle.
- Next take the East corner folding it on an angle toward the top diamond.
- Then take the West corner and fold it along the same angle toward the opposite side. This should make the shape of a flower bud.
- Lastly fold the bottom South triangle under to make a straight line where the stem will be inserted.
- The second part is making the flower stem. Begin again with the white side of the paper facing up and the decorative side on the table.
- Make sure the paper is in a diamond shape facing you.
- Fold the paper in half making a vertical crease down the center.
- Open the paper back up so that it is flat on the table.
- Take the East side and fold the edge of the paper down the center crease just created.
- Next take the West side and fold it to meet in the center line as well.
- Then fold the two sides together creating an elongated triangle which will become the stem of the flower.

- Lastly fold the bottom of the stem so that it is flat and able to stand. This will also create a leaf on the stem.
- Finally attach the flower bud to the stem.

Variation: There are plenty of other variations of how to make a rose using crepe paper or tissue paper depending on how complicated the art therapist would like the art making portion of the session to be. I have also facilitated this directive simply drawing or water coloring a flower and integrating writing the rose, thorn, bud into the image.

Description: Symbolic Goodbye

Supplies: Water-Soluble Paper, Wishing Paper, or other Disappearing Style Papers, Washable Markers, Pencils, Erasers, and a Large Clear Bowl of Water

Directions: There are a number of different products that disappear by burning, dissolving, or floating away that can provide the symbolic example of something ending. I personally prefer the water-soluble disappearing paper because of ease in a therapeutic setting. Ask the client to think of something they have worked through or would like to say goodbye to from their therapeutic work (i.e. dependence on substances, need to be perfect, past trauma). The therapist can also do the same about something the client has overcome in their work together.

Variation: I learned this technique from a colleague friend at New York Presbyterian. For ending on-going therapeutic groups, the disappearing water-soluble paper works well because group members can write something on the paper in various colored washable markers and as they place the paper into the larger clear bowl of water, the colors will wash off and eventually become one beautiful combined new color all together.

Chapter 28

Trauma

Art herapy has become known as a treatment of choice for helping to heal past trauma. There is more research available in this area of our work than in any other subfield. Traumas can occur through medical health emergencies, sudden losses, abuse, neglect, sexual violence, or natural disaster. As many art therapists work in in-patient hospital settings, we see a high number of patients who have experienced one or multiple past traumas. I have worked with those healing from past trauma on varying levels of care including in-patient hospitals, residential treatment centers, outpatient care, private practice, and a student center at the university where I work. What astounds me the most is the resilience of people. I recall a statistic from one of the in-patient hospitals I worked at that at least 80% of patients at the hospital level of care had experienced trauma. Outdated treatment modalities for trauma used to include retelling in detail the traumatic experience to a therapist or psychiatrist, which we now know is not beneficial and potentially re-traumatizing. We experience and store trauma in the body, and therefore, an expressive modality that engages both the brain and body can help process these past experiences in a gentler way. Not only is visual art therapy an effective therapeutic modality, but all of the creative arts – music, dance movement, drama, and expressive writing – are proven beneficial. Below are a variety of art therapy directives that are particularly helpful for working on past trauma.

Further Reading: A well-encompassed compilation book about art therapy and trauma is *Art Therapy, Trauma, and Neuroscience: Theoretical and Practical Perspectives* edited by Juliet L. King (2016).

Description: Bi-Lateral Drawing

Supplies: Large Sheet of Drawing Paper 24" × 36", Painter's or Making Tape, Oil Pastels, Chalk Pastels, or Markers

Directions: I attended Cornelia Elbrecht's *Guided Drawing as Bilateral Body Mapping for Healing Trauma* (2018) training through the Expressive Therapies Summit where I learned the basics of this technique. I highly recommend

DOI: 10.4324/9781003413363-28

reading the book or attending a training before trying to utilize this technique with clients. Bi-lateral drawing or working with both hands, connects both sides of the brain which can intern aid in emotional processing and regulation and this is especially helpful with past trauma. I generally begin with some basic psycho education about bi-lateral drawing and the benefits for those who have experienced past trauma. Start with the large sheet of paper taped down to the table which is an important step since the eyes will be closed and pressure applied to the surface. Next have the client select their medium and color to work with. Ask the client to either close their eyes or avert their gaze away from the paper. We want to be in a sensory feeling place, not concerned with the image that is created. Using both hands have the client create an upside down "L" shape moving away from the body in a repetitive motion. It is important to start from the center core and move outward in a repetitive motion. The client is free to switch material and shapes throughout the process, following their own intuition and sensory desires. Guide the client to think about where in their body they need healing and what would be soothing for this as they portray this on the paper in front of them. The beauty about this technique is that processing of the past experience is not necessary, this has more of a focus on healing and self-soothing than verbally processing or exploring the past trauma, which we now know can be re-triggering and not necessarily beneficial.

Further Reading: For more in-depth study in facilitating this technique I recommend *Healing Trauma with Guided Drawing: A Sensorimotor Art Therapy Approach to Bilateral Body Mapping* by Cornelia Elbrecht. Elbrecht also has a training center called The Institute for Sensorimotor Art Therapy and provides various courses.

Description: Boundaries Exploration

Supplies: Watercolor Paper, Watercolor Paints, Watercolor Brushes, Paper Towels, Water Cup, White Crayon or Oil Pastel

Directions: For clients that have experienced trauma, many times a boundary has been crossed. And for some who have endured more than one trauma or repeated offenses, identifying healthy boundaries can become difficult or confusing. For this art therapy directive, clients can explore boundaries through creating a watercolor resist. Have the client begin with white crayon on watercolor paper. Then for the second step they can use watercolor to explore the resistance of the two mediums. There is something remarkable about watching the boundaries becoming so clear as the watercolor is applied to the initial crayon drawing.

Description: Kintsugi

Supplies: Broken Ceramic Bowls, Kintsugi Kit (Epoxy Adhesive, Gold Powder, Application Brushes)

Directions: Kintsugi is the Japanese art of repairing broken clay vessels with gold adhesive to highlight the imperfections. The symbolism for finding beauty in our repaired parts is a beautiful one. I have facilitated this art therapy directive in a trauma focused art therapy group. We began by gathering a few choices of used bowls from a local consignment shop. Next we placed the bowls in a canvas bag and smashed them as a release. Lastly we used the Kintsugi technique to repair the vessels and add beauty to it. Kintsugi supply kits can be purchased online or in art supply stores.

Description: Soothing Stone Coping Skill

Supplies: White Air Dry Clay (Model Magic® is my preference for this project), Markers, and Essential Oils

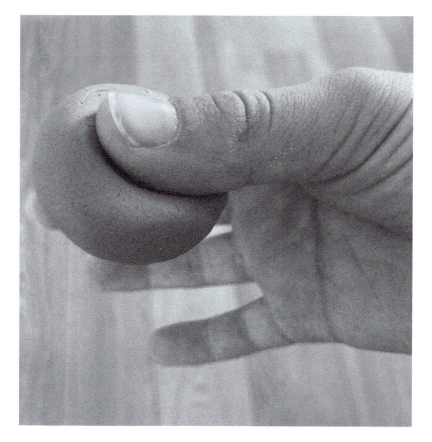

Figure 28.1 Clay Soothing Stone.

Source: Photograph by the author and artwork by Will Balascio.

Directions: When working with clients and groups focused on healing from past trauma, I find it important to explore coping skills. I begin this session with psycho education around triggers and coping skills. Being triggered after trauma is most likely inevitable, so having readily accessible coping skills for this is essential. I generally bring a handout with a long list of coping skills for group members to keep. One main focus of the coping skills is sensory related tools. This art therapy directive focuses particularly on the sense of touch and smell. In this session, clients will learn to create a clay "soothing stone" that can be kept nearby for when they may feel distressed. Therefor the act of creating it is soothing and the end product is also a coping mechanism. Begin by having the client warm up the clay. They can add color with washable markers and essential oil if they desire. Next roll the clay into a small ball after coloring it and adding the aroma. Lastly, press down gently between two fingers into the shape of a finger indentation. Once hardened, this can be a small soothing item to be kept in the client's pocket or other easily accessible spot.

Contraindicated: As mentioned previously some people have a stronger sensitivity to smell, and the use of essential oils would not be recommended.

Reference List

Elbrecht, C. (2018). *Healing trauma with guided drawing: A sensorimotor art therapy approach to bilateral body mapping*. Berkeley, CA: North Atlantic Books.

King, J. (2016). *Art therapy, trauma, and neuroscience: Theoretical and practical perspectives*. New York, NY: Routledge.

Chapter 29

Veterans & First Responders

Nurses, Doctors, Emergency Medical Technicians, Fire Fighters, Police Officers, and Armed Services professionals are all vocations where thinking quickly and acting calmly in the face of a crisis are essential. However, witnessing trauma after trauma and stuffing it away can take a toll on a person, sometimes leading to post-traumatic stress. Veterans and first responders have a tendency to think of others before themselves and can put off getting help. Organizations like The Armed Services Arts Partnership aim to help these individuals through the arts: music, drama, writing, and visual art. Much research has been done by James Pennebaker and C. K. Chung (2011) on the benefits of expressive writing on veterans transitions from the military, noting that "expressive writing holds promise for improving health and functioning among veterans experiencing reintegration difficulty." I have been privileged to work with both student veterans and veterans transitioning from the military to civilian life at the university where I work. I have witnessed firsthand the ease that writing and creativity can give when sharing about the challenges that come with these emergency professions. The COVID-19 pandemic put front-line medical workers under a great deal of stress, being short-staffed, and witnessing an unimaginable amount of loss. These professionals have also suffered post-traumatic stress, and I think, unfortunately, we will continue to see the effects of the pandemic on these professionals in the years to come. While many of these professionals have suffered trauma, the art therapy directives below are more specific to working with veterans and first responders.

Further Reading: For a more in-depth look at working with military professionals specifically I suggest *Art Therapy with Veterans* edited by Rachel Mims (2021).

Description: Art Journaling

Supplies: Blank Journals, Pencil, Eraser, Colored Pencil, Pens, Fine Point Permanent Marker, Collage Magazines and Scrap Paper, Scissors, and Glue Sticks

DOI: 10.4324/9781003413363-29

Directions: Art journaling is the combination of art making and writing. When I have clients who may be tentative about beginning art making, I have found this to be a useful tip-toe into the arts. Depending on the client and their needs, you can simply give them the materials and let them lead with jumping right in. However, if the client needs more direction I will give broad topics for them to focus on. In the past, I have used some of the below prompts when working with veterans and first responders:

- Today I am Feeling
- Visual Bucket List
- Some Thing Holding Me Back
- Gratitude List

Video: This directive can also be explained through a video format. Please see https://www.youtube.com/watch?v=BIusCUUViJo&t=882s for a video explanation on the William & Mary Health and Wellness YouTube.

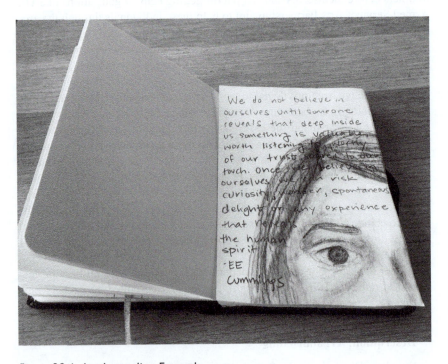

Figure 29.1 Art Journaling Example.

Source: Photograph and artwork by the author.

Description: Expressive Writing

Supplies: Lined or Blank Journals, Pencil, Eraser, Colored Pencil, Markers, or Watercolor Pencils, Watercolor Brushes, Water Cup and Paper Towel

Directions: Expressive writing is a well known therapeutic modality for veterans different than art journaling. Expressive writing has more of a focus on creative writing rather than mixed media art making. However I usually encourage clients to create a small image or doodle to go along with the written piece. Below are some prompts I have used in working with veterans:

• Share an experience from your career that you are most proud of
• What is your favorite quote and why is meaningful to you
• I come from… I am going to
• What is the best advice you were ever given and did you take it

Description: Happy Place

Supplies: Canvas, Acrylic Paint, Paint Palette, Paint Brushes, Water Cup, and Paper Towels

Directions: When your career is highly stressful like a medical professional, first responder, or armed service employee, it can be helpful to take small breaks in the day to meditate or use positive visualization. A classic for many people is to visualize their "happy place." For this art therapy directive, ask clients to begin with a brief meditation and visualization about their personal happy place. This could be an actual place they have traveled to, a cozy spot in their home, or with a pet or loved one. Next have the client create a painting realistic or abstract to represent this. Clients can keep this in their work space, locker, or other break room area as a reminder.

Description: Shame Off You

Supplies: Drawing Paper, Pencil, Eraser, Colored Pencils, Chalk or Oil Pastels

Directions: Shame is an unpleasant but common feeling that we may have made a mistake or done something wrong and because of this we are embarrassed or feeling not good enough. Bene Brown's legendary book *Daring Greatly: How the Courage to Be Vulnerable Transforms the Way We Live, Love, Parent, and Lead* focuses on the emotion of shame. Brown (2012) says "Shame cannot survive being spoken. It cannot tolerate having words wrapped around it. What it craves is secrecy, silence, and judgement." Often veterans or other front line workers may feel an unwarranted sense of shame due to some of their past work experiences. Looking at these feelings of shame is an important way to release it and take its power away. For this art therapy

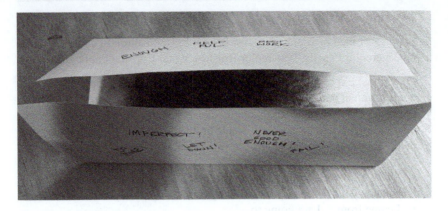

Figure 29.2 Shame Off You Drawing.
Photograph and artwork by the author.

directive, begin by having the client think about what shame feels like and abstractly create that on the paper. For the second step, have the client fold that paper into thirds. Next, ask them to write the words or phrases that come into their mind regarding shame or the circumstance around it. Lastly on the third folded layer, have the client write opposing words or phrases. An example could be "I could have done more to help" and the opposing phrase would be "I have saved many people." We begin by recognizing the feeling in our body, tracing the thoughts that come with it, then reframing those words to a more truthful experience. The layering and steps involved in this art therapy directive are what can help the client explore their thoughts around shame.

Reference List

Brown, B. (2012). *Daring greatly: How the courage to be vulnerable transforms the way we live, love, parent, and lead*. New York, NY: Avery.

Mims, R. (Ed.) (2021). *Art therapy with veterans*. London: Jessica Kingsley Publishers.

Pennebaker, J. W., & Chung, C. K. (2011). *Expressive writing and its links to mental and physical health. Oxford Handbook of health psychology*. Oxford: Oxford University Press.

Chapter 30

Warm Ups & Creative Exploration

A favorite quote of mine by Albert Einstein is, "Creativity is contagious, pass it on." Prior to working at the College of William & Mary's McLeod Tyler Wellness Center, I had mainly worked in acute care settings. It has been an interesting turn in my career as an art therapist to explore creativity from a prevention standpoint. I like to compare art making to daily practices of yoga, meditation, breathwork, or any other wellness exercise. I work with students, faculty, and staff on creativity as a means of self-expression, stress reduction, mindfulness, and general well-being. Most people come into art therapy with reluctance around "not being an artist." Some people haven't done art since elementary school, which is a crying shame! Somewhere along the line, we shift art into a different category than other educational subjects. We cannot expect ourselves to still be a skilled artist without doing it for years. I have not taken any classes on engineering, and therefore, I could never expect myself to be an engineer! People tend to think that you either "are or are not" an artist, as if we are either born with a talent or not. I love to debunk this myth, especially with the most hesitant participants. It is just a matter of practicing art making, just like any other skill that takes training, such as learning a foreign language or playing a musical instrument. The more you make art, the better you will be at it. Additionally, art therapy focuses on the process and the experience for the participant, not the end product. I have led art therapy sessions for general well-being but also for team building, which the art therapy directives below work well for. They are also valuable introductory exercises for a new or reluctant art therapy client.

Description: Finish this Drawing

Supplies: Drawing Paper, Black Marker, Pencil, Colored Pencil or Markers

Directions: For this art therapy directive clients use their creativity to turn a pre-made line into a realistic drawing. This art therapy directive is best in a group format, but if working individually both the therapist and the client should create their own piece since the most interesting part is comparing what each person can create from the same beginning line.

DOI: 10.4324/9781003413363-30

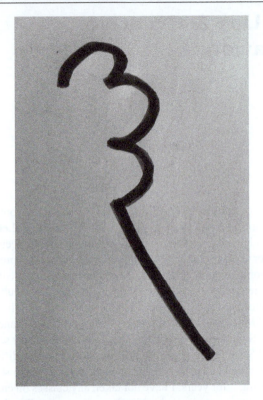

Figure 30.1 Finish This Drawing Example Starter Line.

Source: Photograph and artwork by the author.

Variation: This is a particularly good directive for virtual art therapy sessions. I usually share on the screen the starting line drawing. Next the group participants recreate it on their own paper at home before turning it into a complete drawing and sharing at the conclusion of the session.

Description: Inside/Outside Masks

Supplies: Cardboard Masks, Permanent Markers, Acrylic Paint, Paint Palette, Paint Brushes, Water Cup, Tissue Paper, Magazines, Scissors, Glue Sticks, Decoupage Glue and Brush (Mod Podge® is my preference for this project)

Directions: I like to use this introductory art therapy directive at the start of a new but on-going group. Using cardboard or paper mâché masks, ask clients to think about who they are and what they portray to the world. Paper Mache masks can be purchased in bulk online or in craft supply stores. On the

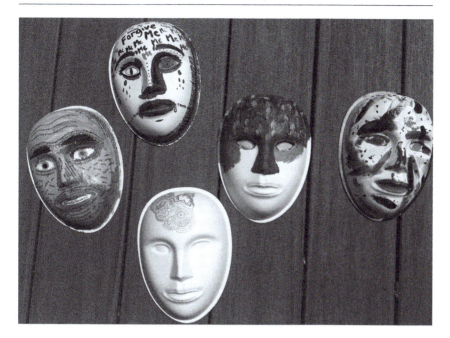

Figure 30.2 Paper Mache Mask Examples.

Source: Photograph by the author.

outside of the mask, clients can portray either abstractly or realistically who they present on the outside. For the inside of the mask, ask clients to go a little deeper and represent more what they are like on the inside or what might take others a little longer to get to know them.

Description: Scribble Drawing

Supplies: Drawing Paper, Black Marker, Pencil, Eraser, Colored Pencil or Markers

Directions: Perhaps the most well known and classic art therapy directive is the scribble drawing. It is said to be that Florence Cane, one of the pioneers of art therapy, created this intervention (Cane, 1983). I was first introduced to this art therapy intervention in my graduate program at Pratt Institute. This art therapy directive is good for getting hesitant participants to begin the process of art making. It is also helpful for those looking to be creative briefly, but are in need of inspiration maybe as a daily practice. I begin the session, by explaining to clients that we will be making an image from a scribbled line. This tends to take the pressure off reluctant participants because I assure them that it will always turn out a little wonky and not exactly right because it began from a scribble. I ask clients to either close their eyes or avert their gaze and make a scribble using the black marker on paper. This line could be wavy, zig zag, curved whatever they feel like. Next, I have the client sit quietly with the scribble turning in various directions until they see something realistic they could turn it into. Participants then use pencil to add the supplementary necessary lines to make it into this object. While many times in art therapy we stray away from abstract, for this exercise I encourage clients to make something realistic. After adding the pencil marks to the original scribble, clients can add color to their picture. I like using the black marker on the initial line because that way we can easily see where they started from.

Variation: When working with a group, ask participants to make a scribble and then pass it to the person next to them to create the image from.

Description: Surreal Collage

Supplies: Magazines, Old Calendars or Posters, Scissors, and Glue Sticks

Directions: When starting a new group or with clients reluctant about art making, collage is a good medium to start off with. Collage tends to be less intimidating because it is mainly about arranging images that are already created. This particular excise is also helpful because it gives the client a place to start from since beginning a creation is often one of the hardest parts. In this art therapy directive, the art therapist will need to pre-select the larger background image to work on top of. I usually have a file folder on hand with some of these readily available. I typically pick backgrounds that are at least the size of a standard magazine page. In general, I pick backgrounds either indoors or outside but with minimal words on the page. The more interesting or unusual the better! I also usually keep old wall calendars for this purpose as well. If working individually, offer the client three or so choices to pick as a background. If working with a group, I like to place one background at each person's spot with maybe a handful of additional options to swap out if necessary in the center of the table. I then introduce the idea of surrealist art to the group or client. Surrealism is a movement in art that means 'above reality' (The Tate Museum, 2023). The images are often believed to be from the unconscious or dream-like and can be wildly bizarre. This idea of strange or wild images can be a way of reducing intimidation in the art making process because it is far from realistic. Working from the background, ask the client to create a picture that tells a story. I also suggest clients stay away from words and mostly focus on images. I always let clients know that this image does not necessarily mean anything about them nor will be analyzed in anyway. However, I do have clients share their piece and often ask if there is anything *they* can relate to in the image.

Reference List

Cane, F. (1983). *The artist in each of us*. Craftsbury Common, VT: Art Therapy Publications.

The Tate Museum. (2023). *Surrealism*. Retrieved from https://www.tate.org.uk/art-terms/s/surrealism.

Chapter 31

Virtual Art Therapy

We were all quickly thrust into virtual art therapy sessions and other forms of telehealth in March of 2020, when COVID-19 disrupted all of our lives. Sadly, the global pandemic cost many lives and left us in a wake of grief and trauma. However, one element that came to light is how we communicate and connect with one another virtually. Within weeks, I was learning new skills and transferred art therapy sessions at the university and eating disorder treatment center where I was working at the time to online. As time grew longer and longer with the global pandemic, we realized we would need more skills to continue our work for an extended period of time. It began to feel limiting by the materials people would have available to them at home rather than a full offering, like in a typical art therapy studio. Being creative with at-home mediums or figuring out means to get them to clients and patients became essential. More and more has been evolved from this time period in terms of digital developments as well as access to at-home materials. In general, I have found the web site The Therapist Aid (2023), developed by Woody Schuldt, a Licensed Mental Health Counselor, to be a great resource for free virtual resources and tools. Below are some virtual art therapy directives and techniques that I found were particularly successful, as well as some effective computer applications that I have utilized with clients.

Further Reading: For an excellent edited collection book with numerous resources on this topic I suggest, *Virtual Art Therapy* edited by Michelle Winkel (2022).

Description: Found Objects Art

Supplies: Computer (or other similar device), Internet Access, Tele-Health Application, and Household Objects

Directions: I thought of this creative, virtual activity when the pandemic first started and we quickly had to pivot to online with minimal access to other outside materials. During this period of time we could not go to stores or even order supplies online. Ask clients to use simple found objects from around their home to create something. For an added challenge, refine this directive

DOI: 10.4324/9781003413363-31

even further limited just to their work space. The challenge is to transform these random household objects into an actual other thing. Often art therapy directives are open ended and many times abstract, but for this exercise I encourage clients to make something realistic not abstract. I have seen sticky notes turned into origami paper cranes and paper clips molded and shaped into a facial profile. The object of this directive is to be creative, resilient, and think outside the box.

Description: Group Mandala

Supplies: Computer (or other similar device), Internet Access, Tele-Health Application, Drawing Paper Cut into Circles, Pencil, Eraser, Colored Pencils, Pens, Fine Point Markers, Watercolor Pencils, Watercolor Brushes, Water Cup, and Paper Towels

Directions: Similar to creating a traditional mandala, however this art therapy directive works best in a group and in a virtual session. Each participant has their own paper circle in front of them and various types of drawing materials. Often mandalas are started in the center and working outward, but in this exercise clients can create anywhere they choose to inside the circle. Going around one at a time, each participant will direct the group members what to draw. For example, a participant could say "draw a small circle inside a larger square in any two opposite colors." In the end comparing the mandalas is interesting because they all contain the same elements but many look very different.

Description: Virtual Round Robin

Supplies: Computer (or other similar device), Internet Access, Tele-Health Application, Drawing Paper, Pencil, Eraser, Markers, or Colored Pencils

Directions: I learned this collaborative art therapy directive in my graduate program at Pratt Institute and adapted it into a virtual exercise. The traditional exercise is in Chapter 12: Group Rapport. Participants each direct one another with something to draw on their paper. An example could be, "draw something in the sky." However rather than passing your paper around the room, group members can each decide on a different prompt for each round while working on their own paper at home. Similarly comparing these drawings during the processing portion of the group is very interesting since they all have the same elements but may be put together completely differently.

Description: Virtual Sand Tray

Supplies: Computer (or other similar device), Internet Access, and a Tele-Health Application

Directions: While not technically art therapy, sand play work is closely related. I was afforded the opportunity to learn about this specialty in my graduate art therapy program at Pratt Institute in a course taught by an expert in sand play and skilled art therapist mentor Josie Abbenante. I recommend at least a continuing education course in sand play before trying this modality otherwise it might not be as affective for the client. Virtual sand play is not exactly the same as touching the sand and manipulating the small items, but is a useful and interesting exploration when working virtually. There are a few online sand tray web sites and programs but my recommended web site is www.onlinesandtray.com developed by Dr. Karen Fried and is free to use (Online Sand Tray, 2023). Thank you to my close friend and clinician Meghan for this recommendation.

Reference List

Online Sand Tray. (2023). *Online Sand Tray by Dr. Karen Fried*. Retrieved from https://www.onlinesandtray.com.
The Therapist Aid. (2023). *Essential Tools for Mental Health Professionals*. Retrieved from https://www.therapistaid.com.
Winkel, M. (2022). *Virtual Art Therapy*. New York, NY: Routledge.

Chapter 32

Conclusion

The practice of art therapy has greatly expanded in recent years, and it has been shown to be extremely valuable in helping individuals and groups in a variety of therapeutic settings. Many art therapists work in hospitals or other clinical settings where they see clients and patients with a wide variety of ages, diagnoses, or therapeutic goals. Additionally, most art therapists will have more than one job in their lifespan and therefore work in various types of settings. This leads to art therapists needing a broad depth of knowledge about many types of clients and their therapeutic goals. In facilitating group or individual sessions, art therapists often use art therapy directives in their work to help clients work on or explore a particular therapeutic goal and the use of a particular art medium. Art therapy directives are clinical directions for a particular session and often require the use of specific art media, both of which are tailored to the client's particular need in the moment by the trained art therapist. As trained art therapists, we are often looking for new directives or to build a collection of them to have available as practitioners to refer to for various client needs. This was even specifically requested by a fellow art therapist on a professional social media group and echoed by others, which inspired this book.

The current resources available to assist trained art therapists in selecting art therapy directives are limited. Numerous art therapy books have been written for use with different populations. These resources are typically written for art therapists working with a specific population, and they explore the underlying diagnoses in great depth with sometimes limited space devoted to art therapy directives. The trained art therapist therefore has to scour numerous resources in developing directives for their practice. There is not one comprehensive guide where directives can be found for use with various populations or with a range of themes and art mediums, and this was my goal with this book that I hope to have fulfilled.

As stated earlier, my intention with this book is not to simply give exacting templates to new art therapists or other mental health professionals. It is in fact the opposite to organize and make available art therapy directives that may inspire trained clinicians to use as a starting point with their own skill set leading

DOI: 10.4324/9781003413363-32

their work with clients and patients. It is my intention to provide a quick-at-a-glance system where each clinician can then use their specific training and framework to then take a step further. Being the most present as possible with our clients and working from our own framework and internal compass as to what works best.

I have included 30 chapters on various populations, diagnoses, and therapeutic goals, including Adolescents and Young Adults, Anger Management, Anxiety, Autism Spectrum, Children, Depression, Eating Disorders, Emotion Recognition, Eco-Art, Family, Grief, Group Rapport, LGBTQIA+, Life Transitions, Medical, Mindfulness, Multiculturalism, Older Adults and Dementia, Personality Disorders, Pregnancy and Fertility, Psychotic Disorders, Self Esteem, Spirituality, Substance Abuse, Supervision, Termination, Trauma, Veterans and First Responders, Warm Ups and Creative Exploration, and Virtual Art Therapy. This list is not necessarily exhaustive, but I am hopeful it has covered the majority of situations a clinician may be considering. Each chapter has four art therapy directives that fit with the chapter. However, many of these can overlap or be altered to work with different sections of the book. Again, it is up to each clinician to utilize these as best they see appropriate for their particular client, family, or group. Likewise, most of these art therapy directives can be adapted to work for individuals or groups. It is my goal for this book to inspire creativity for clinicians to utilize in their own powerful way.

Lastly, I would like to thank my art therapy community for the inspiration to write this book. While I always knew I wanted to work in the field of visual art, I meandered my way through various art careers until finding art therapy. I began with museum work, an art auction house, and eventually settled on art education. I liked being an art teacher and was confident in my skills to teach various art techniques, but it was not the media techniques that I found most interesting. My attention was drawn to the students who struggled in other classes but found art more doable. I wondered why so many students wanted to come to the art room at recess for "open art" instead of attempting to manage tricky social dynamics on the playground. Despite already having a master's degree in art education and several years of teaching under my belt, I took the leap and went back for a second master's degree in art therapy from Pratt Institute. From the moment I began my first class, it clicked. I was with my people and where I was supposed to be. I am grateful for the learning experience I gained there for me both personally and professionally. Once I completed my degree I felt equipped even in my first job working in the hospital setting of an adolescent mental health unit. So I would like to offer my appreciation to the art therapy program at Pratt Institute for this gift. As I continued on my career path as an art therapist, despite having moved for family reasons a few times, I was fortunate to have remarkable job opportunities wherever we landed. Colleagues at the Brattleboro Retreat and New York Presbyterian were just as much my teachers as my graduate program was, and I keep their skills with me today. I feel so lucky because when people talk about their jobs with boredom or lackluster, I feel the opposite. Every client, patient, family, or group is an exciting opportunity for me to share with them the power of art making and what is possible inside of them. While seemingly intimidating or perhaps the opposite for some too simplistic, most often even the most misbelieving of participants tend to have noticed something within them shift after trying art therapy. I sign my emails with the quote I used above from Albert Einstein, "creativity is contagious, pass it on" because I believe this to be so true. Our work as art therapists should not be sheltered but instead shared.

Index

Note: Page locators in *italics* denote figures.

35 Guided Meditation Scripts: Scripts for Meditation Teachers, Yoga Teachers, Therapists, Coaches, Counsellors and Healers (McWilliam) 63

Abstract Self-portrait 67
Acceptance and Commitment Therapy 80, 86
acrylic 7, 22, 27, 33, 39, 40, 44–45, 47–48, 54, 56, 61–62, 67, 79, 106, 123, 126
adolescents: and art therapy 10–14; Comic Panel 10; Digital Art Altered Self-Portrait 11; Photo Transfer 11–12; Secret Word Mandala 12–14
affirmation journal 98–99
affirmation word 97–98, *98*
Alcoholics Anonymous program 101, 105, 106
altered bookmaking 58–59
American Art Therapy Association (AATA) 3
Anger Container 15
Anger Iceberg 16
anger management: Anger Container 15; Anger Iceberg 16; and art therapy 15–17; Breaking and Rebuilding 16; Stress Ball 16
anxiety: art therapy 18–20; Five Drawings 18–19; Lavender Eye Pillow 19, *20*; Self-Soothing Fidget 19; yoga & art therapy 20
The Armed Services Arts Partnership 121
art: journaling 121–122, *122*; and spirituality 101

Art Psychotherapy 8
art therapy: and adolescents 10–14; advantages of 7–8; and anger management 15–17; anxiety 18–20; Autism Spectrum Disorder 22–25; and children 26–29; cultural considerations 3–4; defined 2; depression 30–33; directives 4–5; eating disorders 34–37; frameworks and styles 8; and grief 50–53; history of 2–3; LGBTQIA+ community 58–61; progression 3–5; and young adults 10–14
Art Therapy, Trauma, and Neuroscience: Theoretical and Practical Perspectives (King) 117
Art Therapy and Childbearing Issues 90
Art Therapy and Healthcare (Malchiodi) 67
Art Therapy and Substance Abuse (Schmanke) 105
Art Therapy with Veterans (Mims) 121
assertiveness training 99–100
Autism Spectrum Disorder: art therapy 22–25; Pillow Stuffed Animal Making 22–23, *23*; Quilling 23–24, *24*; Sensory Sculptures 25; Sensory Tool Kit 25
awe 101–102

Beck, Aaron 107
bi-lateral drawing 117–118
bookmaking 58–59, 98

boundaries exploration 118
Bourgeois, Louis 43
Bracelet Weaving 68–69; diagonal pattern 68; staircase pattern 68–69
Breaking and Rebuilding 16
Brown, Bene 123

Cane, Florence 3, 127
Case Reflection 109–110
Cezanne, Paul 43
Chakras *110*, 110–111
Champagne, Tina 22
Character Strengths and Virtues: A Handbook and Classification (Peterson and Seligman) 80
chalk pastels 6, 20, 48, 49, 73, 117
charcoal 6, *36*, 45, 73, 92, 101, 113
children: and art therapy 26–29; drawing their house 27; Dream Catchers 26–27; Future Self-portrait 27; Power Word 27–29, *28*
Chung, C. K. 121
Clark, Susan M. 86
clay 7, 15, 22, 25, *35*, 37, 39–40, 44, 49, 62–63, 82–83, 90, *91*, 106, 119–120
Clay Coil Pot 82–83
Clay Imprint 90, *91*
Cognitive Behavioral Therapy 80, 86, 107
cognitive distortions 105–106
Collaborative Painting 47–48, *48*
Collaborative Sculpture 38, *39*
collage 6, 11, 25, 34, 58, 79, 100, 103, 112, 128
colored pencil 6, 10, 12, 16, 27, 30–31, 37, 48–49, 51, 56, 58–59, 63, 66, 69, 73–74, 76, 87–88, 92, 94–95, 100–101, 103, 105, 107, 110–111, 113, 121, 123, 125, 127, 131
Comic Panel 10
counter-transference 109
COVID-19 pandemic 6, 121, 130; and art therapists 4
crayons 6, 20, 27, 48–49, 107, 118
Creating a Placemat 34
Creative Arts Therapies and the LGBTQ Community: Theory and Practice (MacWilliam, Harris, Trottier, and Long) 58
Creative Arts Therapy 2
crocheting 7, 34

cultural humility 77
Cultural Humility in Art Therapy: Applications for Practice, Research, Social Justice, Self-Care, and Pedagogy (Jackson) 77

Daring Greatly: How the Courage to Be Vulnerable Transforms the Way We Live, Love, Parent, and Lead (Brown) 123
da Vinci, Leonardo 101
Davis, Barbara Jean 72
DBT-Informed Art Therapy: Mindfulness, Cognitive Behavior Therapy, and the Creative Process (Clark) 86
Decorative Diary Cards *87*, 87–88
dementia 64; and older adults 82–85
depression: art therapy 30–33; Gratitude Tree 31, *32*; HopeFULL 31; Opposite Action 30–31; Portrait by the Art Therapist 33
Diagnostic and Statistical Manual of Mental Disorders 86
diagonal pattern, bracelet weaving 68
Dialectical Behavior Therapy 30–31, 37, 86, 87–89
dialectics 37
Diary Cards 87–88
digital arts 7, 11
Digital Art Altered Self-portrait 11
Dimensions of You Drawing 69
distress tolerance 88
Doll Making 83, *84*
Drawing "Ed" *35*, 37
Drawing From Within: Using Art to Treat Eating Disorders (Hinz) 34
drawing own houses 27
drawings: bi-lateral 117–118; mandala 73; scribble 127–128
drawing to music 94–95
drawing your breath 73
Draw Yourself on a Path 63
Dream Catchers 26–27

eating disorders: art therapy 34–37; Creating a Placemat 34; Drawing "Ed" *35*, 37; knitting blanket 37; Two Opposing Feelings 37
eco-art therapy 38–42; Collaborative Sculpture 38, *39*; Personal

Connection to Nature 39–40; Rock Art 40; Rock Wrapping 40–42, *41*

Eco-Art Therapy in Practice (Pike) 38

Eight Dimensions of Wellness framework 69

Einstein, Albert 125, 135

Elbrecht, Cornelia 117, 118

embroidery 7, 26–27, 50, 68, 83, 98–99

Embroidery Memory 50

Emotion Painting 44

emotion recognition 43–46; Emotion Painting 44; Emotions Character Sculpture 44; Emotions Wheel 44–45; facial expressions 45–46

Emotions Character Sculpture 44

emotions wheel 44–45

Expressive Arts 3

Expressive Therapies Continuum 8

expressive writing 123

facial expressions 45–46

Family Art Psychotherapy: A Clinical Guide And Casebook (Landgarten) 47

family art therapy 47–49; Collaborative Painting 47–48, *48*; Family Portrait 48–49; Favorite Memory 49; genogram 49

Family Portrait 48–49

Farrelly-Hansen, Mimi 101

Favorite Memory 49

Favorite Tunes 83–85

fiber arts 2, 7, 22, 60, *78*, 83

finger knitting 69–70, *70*

Finish this Drawing 125–126, *126*

Five Drawings 18–19

Found Objects Art 130–131

Fried, Karen 132

Future Self-portrait 27, 67

Gateway 113, *114*

Gavron, T. 15

genogram 49

Gift to Yourself 100

Goodbye and Hello 113–115

Gottman, John 16

Gottman, Julie 16

Gratitude Tree 31, *32*

grief 50; and art therapy 50–53; Embroidery Memory 50; Letting

Go Leaf 51, *51–52*; Origami Crane 51–53; Ornament 50–51

Grounding with the Five Senses 94

group art 54–55, *55*

Group Mandala Drawings 73, 131

group rapport 54–57; group art 54–55, *55*; Mini-canvas Collab 56; Round Robin 56; Shapes Match Up 56–57

Growth Printmaking Series 91–92

guided imagery 63–64

Happy Place 123

Harris, B. T. 58

Healing Trauma with Guided Drawing: A Sensorimotor Art Therapy Approach to Bilateral Body Mapping (Elbrecht) 118

Heart and Soul *102*, 102–103

Help for the Helper 111

Heritage Quilt Squares 78–79

higher power 106

Hinz, Lisa 34

HopeFULL 31

hopelessness 31

Hygge 92

Identity Portrait 79

infertility 90–93

Inside Out 44

Inside/Outside Masks 126–127, *127*

Interpersonal Comic 88

I Remember Better When I Paint (Ellena and Huebner) 82

Jackson, Louvenia 77

jewelry making 7, 29

Johansson, B. 82

journaling *65*, 121–123

Kagin, Sandra 8

King, Juliet L. 117

Kintsugi technique 118–119

knitting 7, 34, 37, 68–69, *70*

knitting blanket 37

Kramer, Edith 2, 5

Landgarten, Helen 47

Lavender Eye Pillow 19, *20*

Letting Go Leaf 51, *51–52*

LGBTQIA+ community: Altered Bookmaking 58–59; art therapy 58–61; Pride Buttons *59*, 59–60; Rainbow Yarn Wrapping 60; Song Lyric/Quote 61
life transitions: Acceptance Art 62–63; art therapy 62–66; Draw Yourself on a Path 63; guided imagery 63–64; I Come From *65*, 66
Linehan, Marsha 62, 88
Long, K. 58
Lusebrink, Vija 8

MacWilliam, B. 58
Malchiodi, Cathy 11, 67
Mandala Drawings 12–14, 73, 131
Markers 6, 10, 12, 16, 22, 25, 27, 31, 37, 44, 48–49, 51, 54, 56, 58–59, 63, 73, 78, 83, 85, 87, 90, 94–95, 99–100, 105, 107, 111, 116–117, 119–120, 125–127, 131
masks: Inside/Outside 126–127, *127*; paper mâché 126–127, *127*
materials from nature 7, 38
McWilliam, Susi 63
medical art therapy: Abstract Self-Portrait 67; Bracelet Weaving 68–69; Dimensions of You 69; finger knitting 69–70, *70*
Miller, E. 82
Mims, Rachel 121
Mindful Art Therapy (Davis) 72
mindfulness: Drawing your Breath 73; mandala drawings 73; Mindful *vs.* MindFULL *74*, 74–75; Zendoodles® 76 *75*
Mindful *vs.* MindFULL *74*, 74–75
Mini-Canvas Collab 56
mono printing 95
mosaic tiles 7
multiculturalism 77–80; Heritage Quilt Squares 78–79; Identity Portrait 79; Piece of Me mixed media technique 79, *80*; Values Exploration 79–80
music 3, 8, 22, 67, 73, 79, 83, 85, 94–95, 101, 117, 121, 125

Narcotics Anonymous 105, 106
Naumburg, Margaret 2

negativity 31
nest *92*, 93

oil pastels 6, 37, 92, 100, 117, 123
older adults and dementia 82–85; Clay Coil Pot 82–83; Doll Making 83, *84*; Favorite Tunes 83–85; Velvet Coloring Pages 85
Opposite Action 30–31
origami 51–53, 98, 115, 131
Origami Crane 51–53
ornament, and grief therapy 50–51

painting 6, 40, 44–45, 47–48, *48*, 56, 82, 123
paper mâché masks 126–127, *127*
paper sculptures 7
pencil 6, 10, 12, 16, 18–19, 23–24, 30–31, 33, 37, 48–49, 51, 54, 56, 58–59, 61–63, 66, 69, 73–74, 76, 79, 87–88, 90, 92, 94–95, 97–101, 105–107, 110–111, 113, 115–116, 121, 123, 125, 127–128, 131
Pennebaker, James 121
Personality Disorders 86–89; Decorative Diary Cards *87*, 87–88; distress tolerance 88; Interpersonal Comic 88; Wise Mind 88–89
Peterson, Christopher 80
photo transfer 11–12
Picasso, Pablo 43
Piece of Me mixed media technique 79, *80*
Pike, Amanda Alders 38
Pillow Stuffed Animal Making 22–23, *23*
plaster 7, 106, *107*
Plutchik, Robert 44
portrait 11, 27, 33, 45, 48, 67, 79
Portrait by the Art Therapist 33
Positive Psychology 80
Power Word 27–29, *28*
Pratt Institute 111, 131–132, 134
pregnancy 90–93
Pride Buttons *59*, 59–60
printmaking 91, 95
psychotic disorders 94–96; Drawing to Music 94–95; Grounding with the Five Senses 94; mono printing 95; Watercolor Abstract 95–96, *96*

quilling 23–24, *24*
quilting 6

Radical Acceptance 62–63
Rainbow Yarn Wrapping 60
Rock Art 40
Rock Wrapping 40–42, *41*
Rose, Thorn, Bud activity 115–116
Round Robin 56
Rubin, Judith 3

Safe Haven 106–108, *107*
Schmanke, Libby 105
Schuldt, Woody 130
Scribble Drawing 127–128
sculpture 7, 16, *17*, 25, 38, *39*, 44, 63
Secret Word Mandala 12–14
self-esteem 97–100; Affirmation Journal
    98–99; Affirmation Word 97–98,
    98; Assertiveness Training
    99–100; Gift to Yourself 100
Self-Management and Recovery Training
    105
Self-Soothing Fidget 19
Seligman, Martin 80
Sensory Integration techniques 22
Sensory Sculptures 25
Sensory Tool Kit 25
Shame Off you Drawing 123–124, *124*
Shapes Match Up 56–57
Shella, T. 67
Sholt, M. 15
S.M.A.R.T. 105
song lyric/quote, and art therapy 61
Soothing Stone Coping Skill 119–120
Soul Collage® 103
spirituality 101–103; art and 101; Awe
    101–102; Heart and Soul *102*,
    102–103; Soul Collage® 103;
    Your Creation Story 103
*Spirituality and Art Therapy: Living the
    Connection* (Farrelly-Hansen) 101
staircase pattern, bracelet weaving 68–69
stress ball 16
Styrofoam sheets 91–92
substance abuse and addiction 105–108;
    cognitive distortions 105–106;
    higher power 106; Safe Haven
    106–108, *107*
supervision 109–112; Case Reflection
    109–110; Chakras *110*, 110–111;
    Help for the Helper 111; Vision
    Boards 111–112
surreal collage 128

Swan-Foster, Nora 90
Swarbrick, Peggy 69
Symbolic Goodbye 116

termination 113–116; defined 113;
    Gateway 113, *114*; Goodbye and
    Hello 113–115; Rose, Thorn, Bud
    115–116; Symbolic Goodbye 116
Tervalon, M. 77
The Therapist Aid web site 130
Thyme, K. E. 30
trauma 117–120; Bi-lateral Drawing
    117–118; Boundaries Exploration
    118; Kintsugi technique 118–119;
    Soothing Stone Coping Skill
    119–120
Trottier, D. G. 58
Two Opposing Feelings 37

Ulman, Elinor 3
Ulrich, Roger 38

values clarification 80
values exploration 79–80
Velvet Coloring Pages 85
veterans & first responders 121–124;
    Art Journaling 121–122, *122*;
    Expressive Writing 123; Happy
    Place 123; Shame off you
    Drawing 123–124, *124*
virtual art therapy 130–132; Found Objects
    Art 130–131; Group Mandala 131;
    Virtual Round Robin 131; Virtual
    Sand Tray 131–132
Virtual Art Therapy 130
Virtual Round Robin 131
Virtual Sand Tray 131–132
vision boards 111–112

warm ups & creative exploration 125–129;
    Finish this Drawing 125–126, *126*;
    Inside/Outside Masks 126–127,
    127; Scribble Drawing 127–128;
    Surreal Collage 128
Watercolor Abstract 95–96, *96*
watercolor paints 22, 31, 33, 83, 95, 97,
    102, 106, 110, 113, 118
watercolor pencils 6, 30, 31, 51, 73, 79,
    88, 95, 110, 123, 131
Winkel, Michelle 130
Wise Mind 88–89

women's health 90–93; Clay Imprint 90,
  91; Growth Printmaking Series
  91–92; Hygge 92; Nest *92*, 93

yoga: and anxiety 20; and art therapy 20
young adults: and art therapy 10–14;
  Comic Panel 10; Digital Art

Altered Self-portrait 11; Photo
  Transfer 11–12; Secret Word
  Mandala 12–14
Your Creation Story 103

Zendoodles® 76 *75*

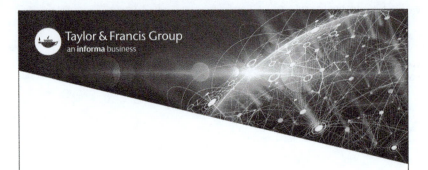

For Product Safety Concerns and Information please contact our EU
representative GPSR@taylorandfrancis.com Taylor & Francis Verlag GmbH,
Kaufingerstraße 24, 80331 München, Germany

Printed and bound by CPI Group (UK) Ltd, Croydon, CR0 4YY
08/06/2025
01897006-0007